‘Grasmere looked so beautiful that my heart was almost melted away.’

Dorothy Wordsworth, *Grasmere Journals*, Saturday 21 June 1800

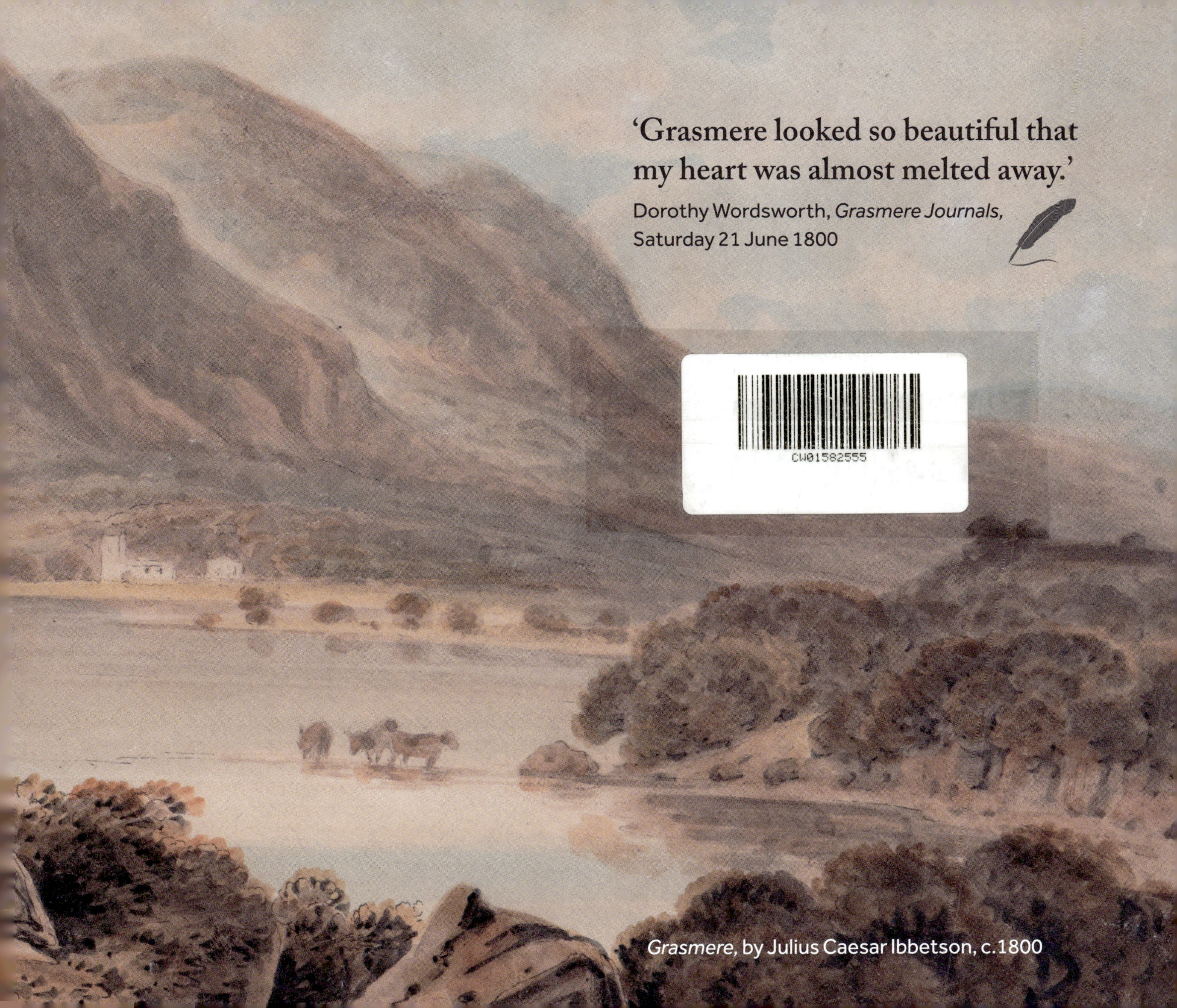

Grasmere, by Julius Caesar Ibbetson, c.1800

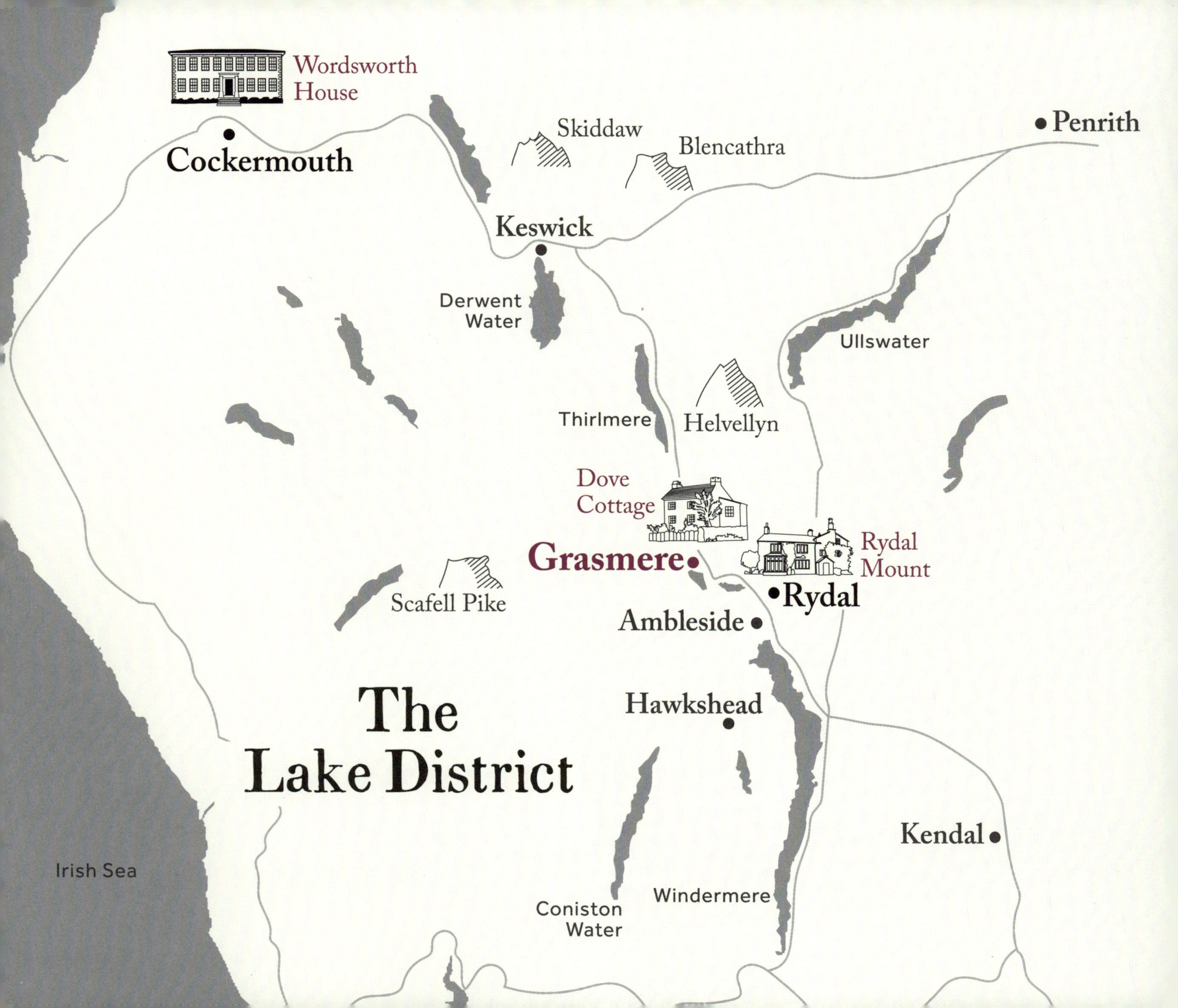
Wordsworth House
Cockermouth
Skiddaw
Blencathra
Penrith
Keswick
Derwent Water
Ullswater
Thirlmere
Helvellyn
Dove Cottage
Grasmere
Rydal Mount
Rydal
Scafell Pike
Ambleside
The Lake District
Hawkshead
Kendal
Irish Sea
Windermere
Coniston Water

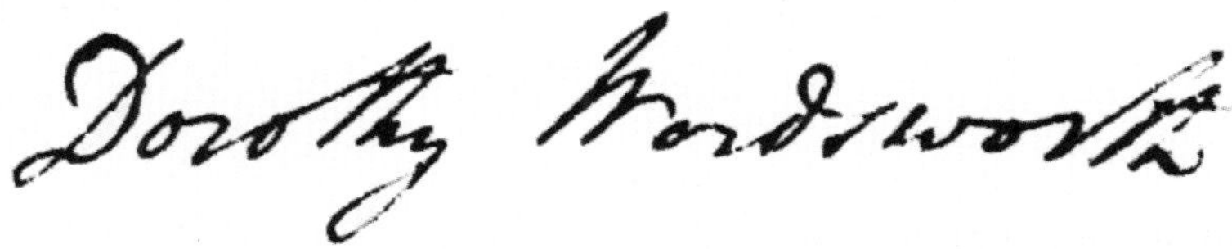

Dorothy Wordsworth's Grasmere Days

Sarah Lawrance

Open Ended Books

A note to the reader

This celebration of the life and writings of Dorothy Wordsworth has been created with the kind assistance of the Wordsworth Trust in Grasmere. Most of the pictures shown in the book are from the Trust's collection. Details of images from other sources are given on page 57.

Where quotations from Dorothy's letters and journals have been included, her spelling and punctuation have been lightly edited for ease of reading.

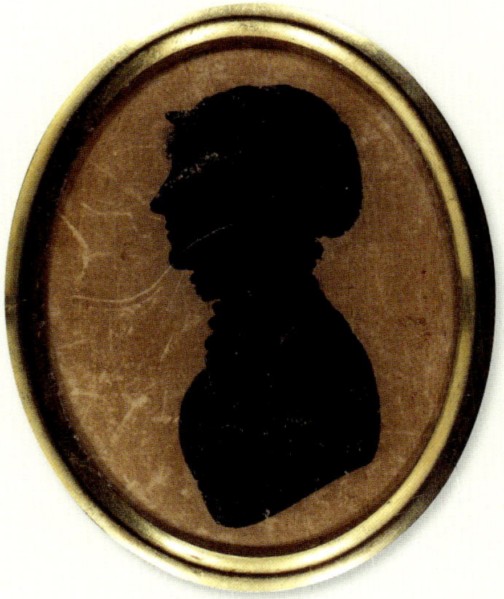

Dorothy Wordsworth (1771–1855), silhouette by an unknown artist, c.1806

'The most wonderful thing is that Dorothy Wordsworth was there and looked about her.'

Pamela Woof, *Dorothy Wordsworth – Wonders of the Everyday,* 2013

Contents

Introducing Miss Wordsworth

Dorothy Wordsworth was the sister of the Romantic poet William Wordsworth. She was also a voracious reader, intrepid hillwalker, loyal friend and prolific writer of letters, journals and poems.

Dorothy's writings reflect her deep care for family, friends and strangers, and her curiosity about the natural world. Her description of climbing Scafell Pike in 1818 is believed to be the earliest such account written by a woman.

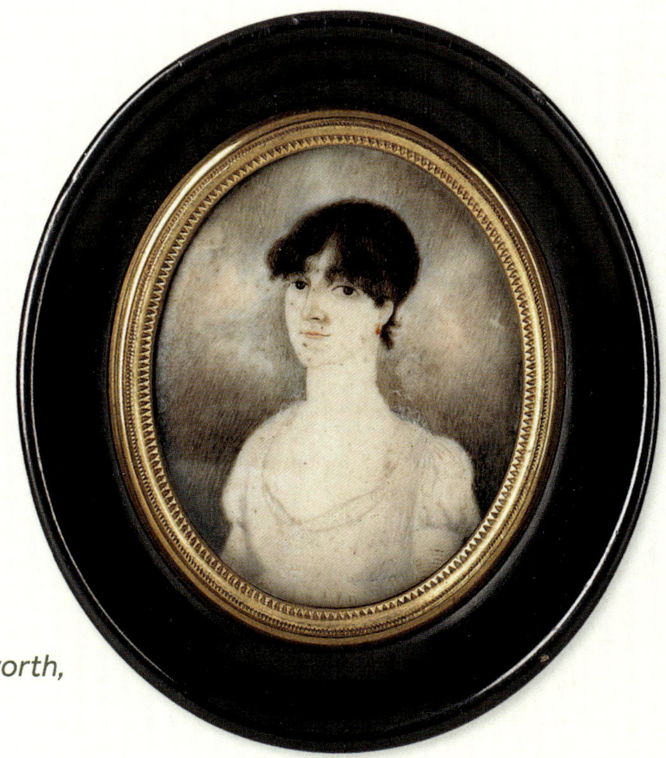

Portrait of a young woman thought to be Dorothy Wordsworth, by an unknown artist, c.1800

Dorothy lived in and around Grasmere for much of her life. Her detailed observations of Lake District landscapes and people inspired some of William's best-known poems.

'She, in the midst of all, preserved me still A Poet...'

William Wordsworth, writing about his sister in his autobiographical poem *The Prelude*, 1805

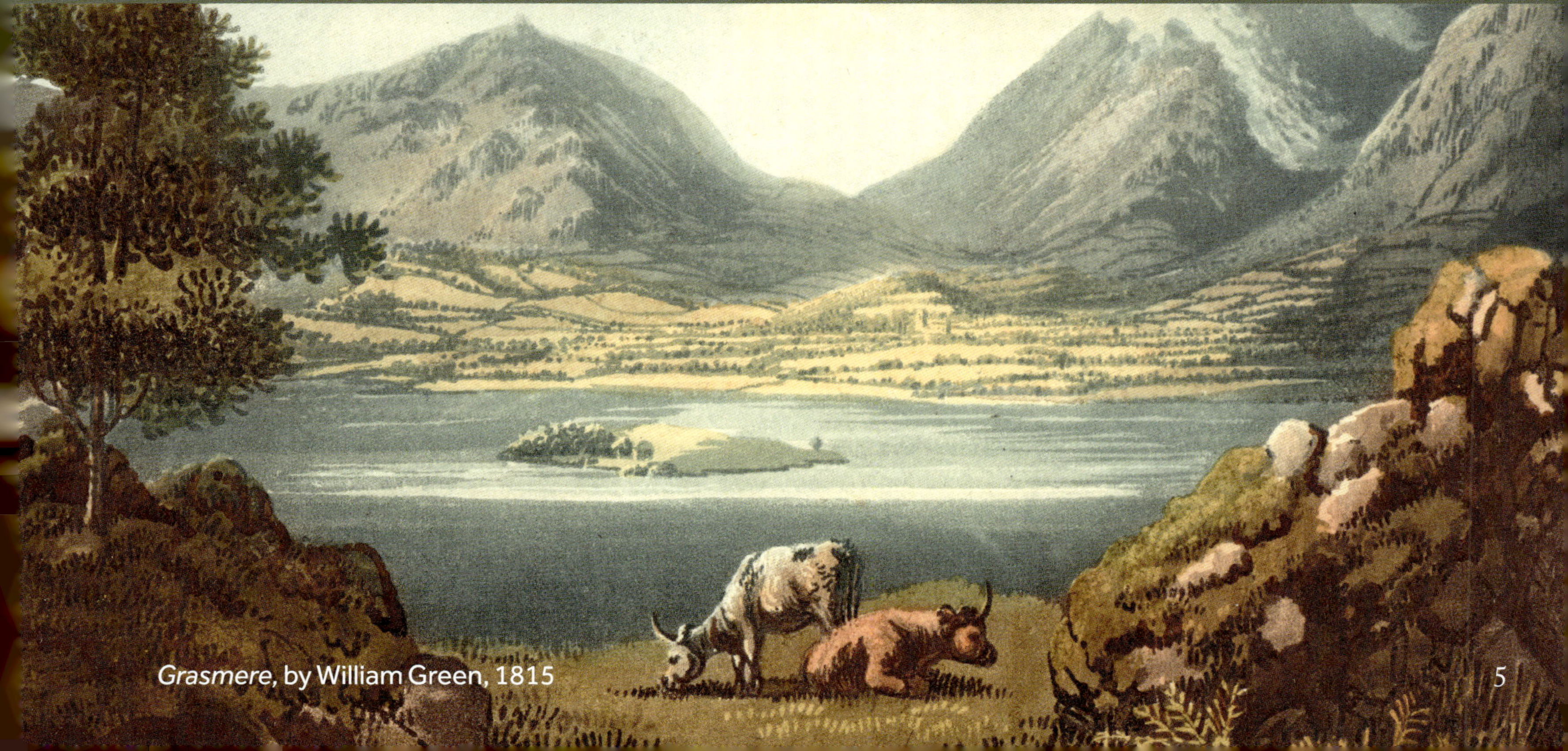

Grasmere, by William Green, 1815

A Christmas baby

Dorothy Wordsworth was born on 25 December 1771, in Cockermouth, on the edge of the Lake District.

Her father, John Wordsworth, was a lawyer, employed by a prominent Cumberland landowner to manage his estates. Dorothy's mother, Ann Cookson, came from nearby Penrith, where her parents ran a haberdashery.

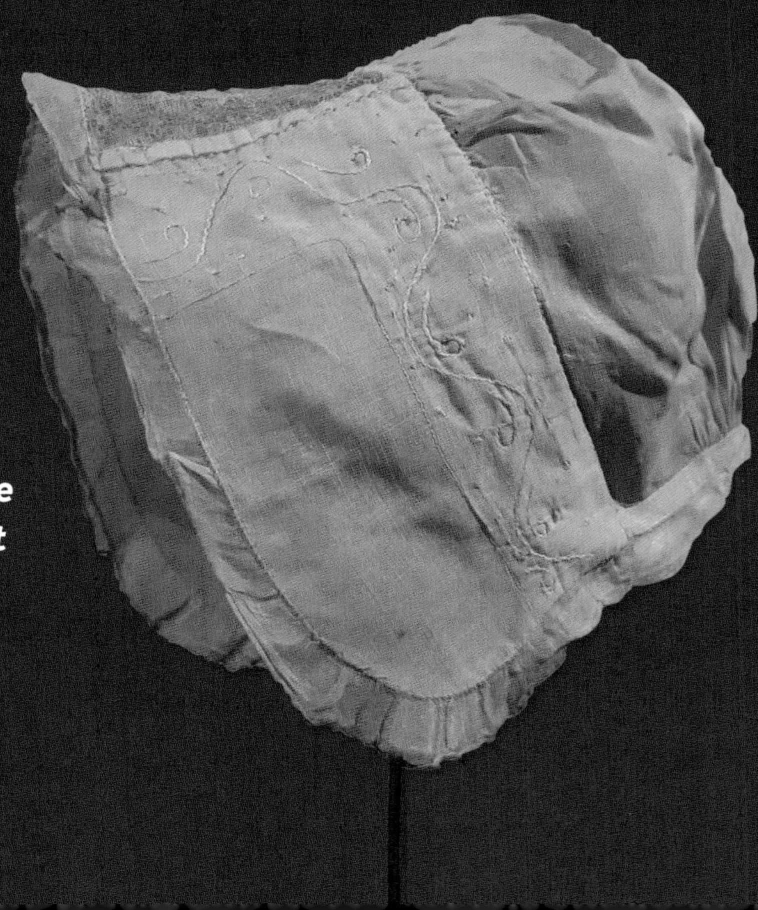

Dorothy Wordsworth wore this beautiful linen bonnet when she was a baby.

Who do you suppose made it for her?

Dorothy was the third of five children, and the only girl. Her brother William was the closest to her in age.

John Wordsworth (1741–1783) *m.* Ann Cookson (1748–1778)

- Richard (1768–1816)
- William (poet) (1770–1850)
- **Dorothy** (1771–1855)
- John (1772–1805)
- Christopher (1774–1846)

This is the imposing house in Cockermouth where Dorothy Wordsworth and her brothers were born. The house did not belong to the Wordsworths – it came rent-free with their father's job.

Etching by E. J. MacWhirter; engraved by H. Manesse, undated

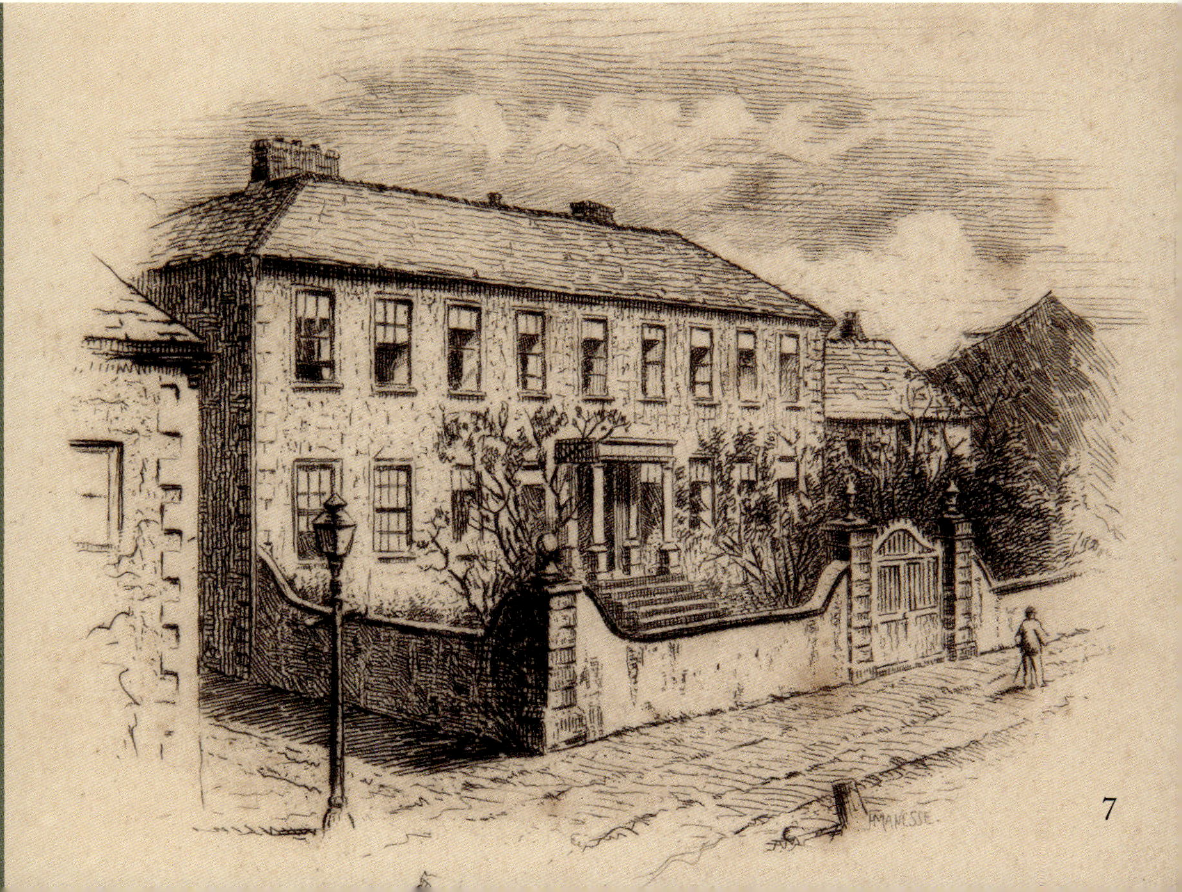

Separated from her brothers... then reunited

When Dorothy Wordsworth was just six years old, her mother died unexpectedly.

Dorothy was sent away to live with relatives in Halifax. She enjoyed school and made lifelong female friends but missed her brothers dearly, William most of all.

When they were reunited, ten years later, Dorothy and William discovered many shared interests, especially reading and poetry.

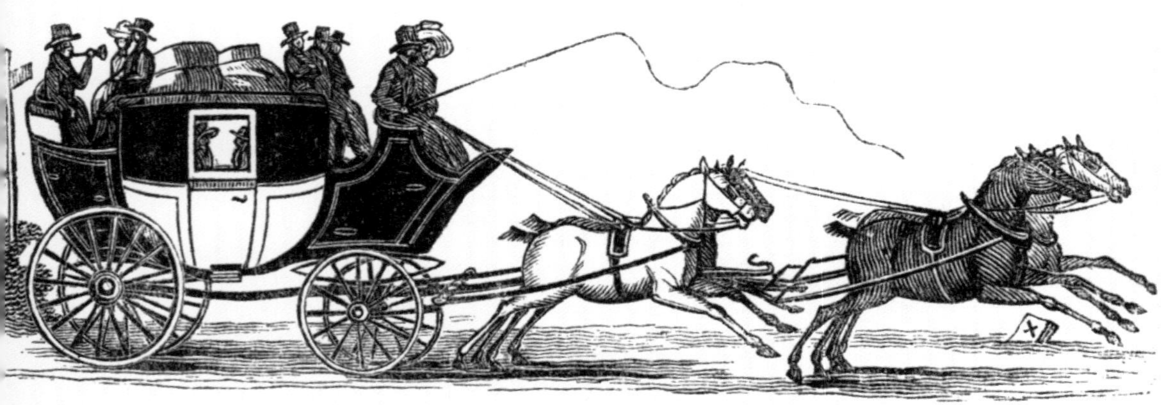

From Cockermouth to Halifax was a journey of some 120 miles by horse and carriage.

How do you think six-year-old Dorothy felt about making this journey?

Dorothy's brothers were sent to school in the little Lake District town of Hawkshead.

After school, William studied at Cambridge University and spent time travelling in Europe. Meanwhile, Dorothy moved from one set of relatives to another, helping with babies and housekeeping.

'I often say to myself, I have the most affectionate brothers in the world…'

Dorothy Wordsworth, Letter to Jane Pollard, 7 August 1787

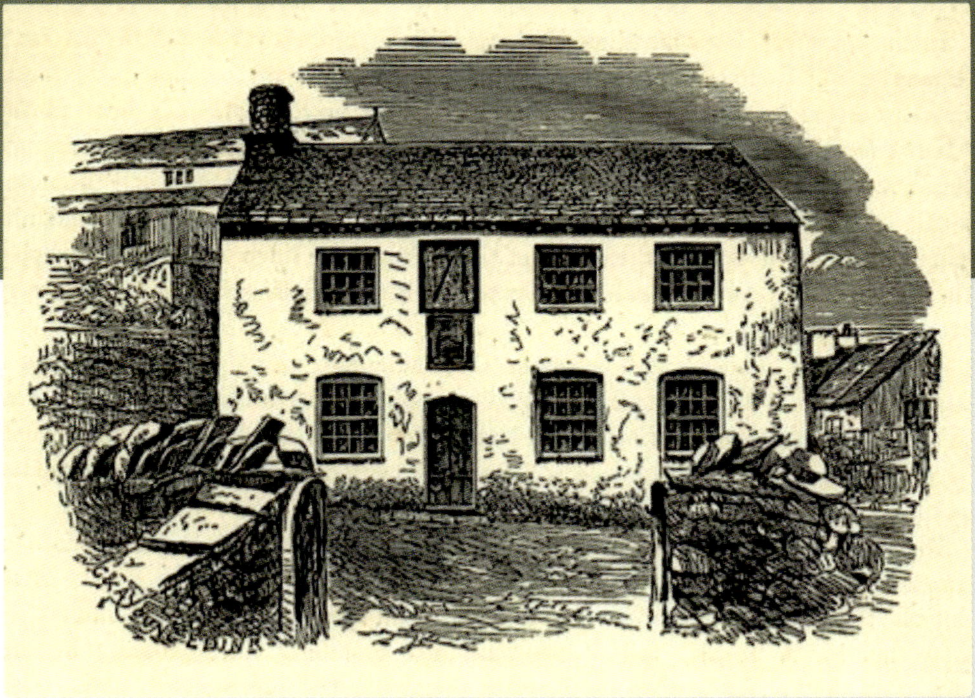

This is the grammar school at Hawkshead, where William and his brothers went to school.

Engraving by C. and A. Young, 1870

Poetry and friendship

Dorothy Wordsworth was determined to support her brother William in his ambition to become a poet.

Dorothy and William became close friends with another young poet, Samuel Taylor Coleridge. With Dorothy's help, in 1798 William and Coleridge published a collection of poems which they called '*Lyrical Ballads*'.

This helped to establish their reputation as two of the foremost poets of their day.

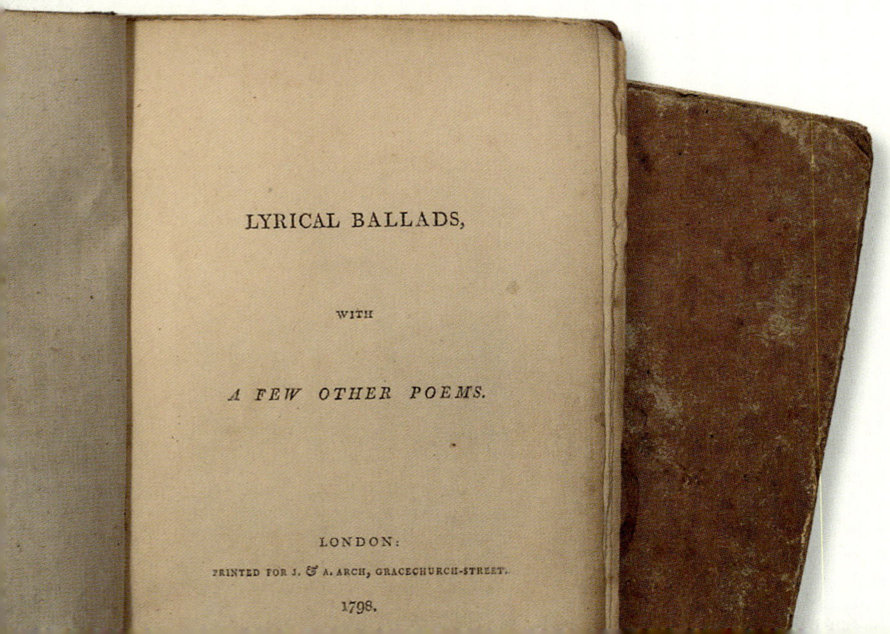

It's hard to believe that this unassuming volume is both famous and valuable.

Would you pick it up if you saw it on the shelf?

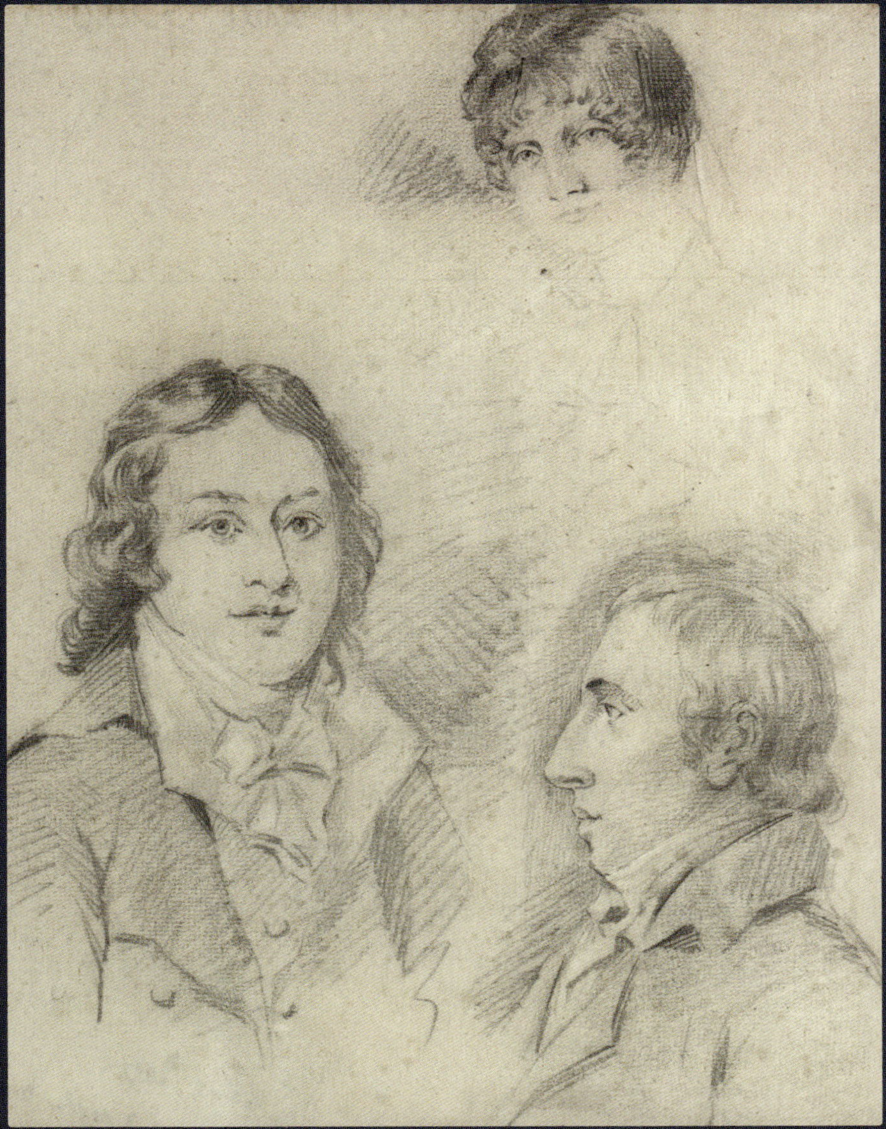

'Coleridge is a wonderful man. His conversation teems with soul, mind and spirit.'

Dorothy Wordsworth, Letter to Mary Hutchinson, June 1797

This is a strange drawing by an unknown artist! The two lower figures are Samuel Taylor Coleridge (left) and William Wordsworth (right).

The woman at the top right is probably Dorothy – but why is her portrait unfinished?

Arriving in Grasmere

After living for several years in the south of England, and briefly in Germany, Dorothy Wordsworth and her brother William returned to the Lake District.

On 20 December 1799 they moved into a small cottage on the edge of Grasmere village. It was nothing fancy, but it became their home for the next eight years, and Dorothy loved it.

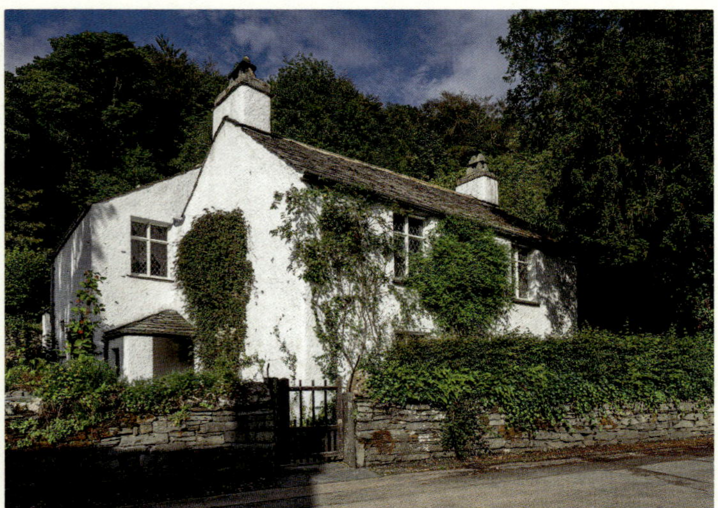

The cottage was once an inn called The Dove and Olive Bough. Today it is known as Dove Cottage.

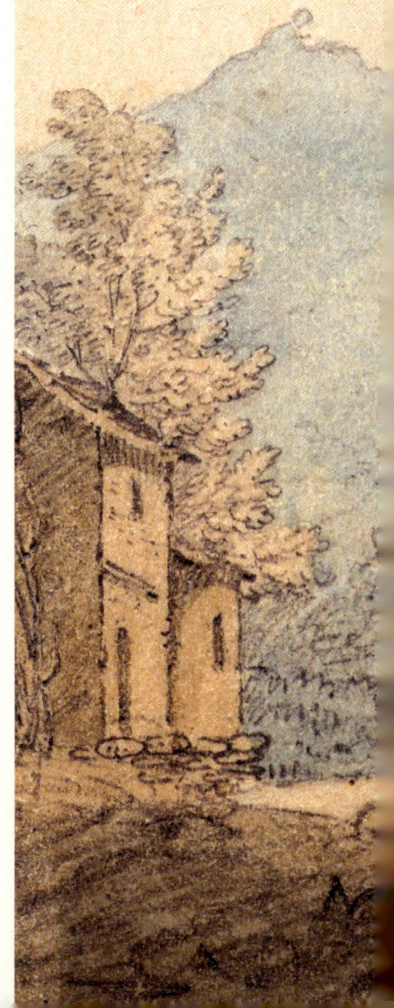

‘We are daily more delighted with Grasmere, and its neighbourhood.’

Dorothy Wordsworth, Letter to Jane Marshall, 10 September 1800

Dorothy told her friend Jane that the cottage was sometimes noisy on account of being so close to the road, but it looks very quiet here.

What noises might she have been talking about?

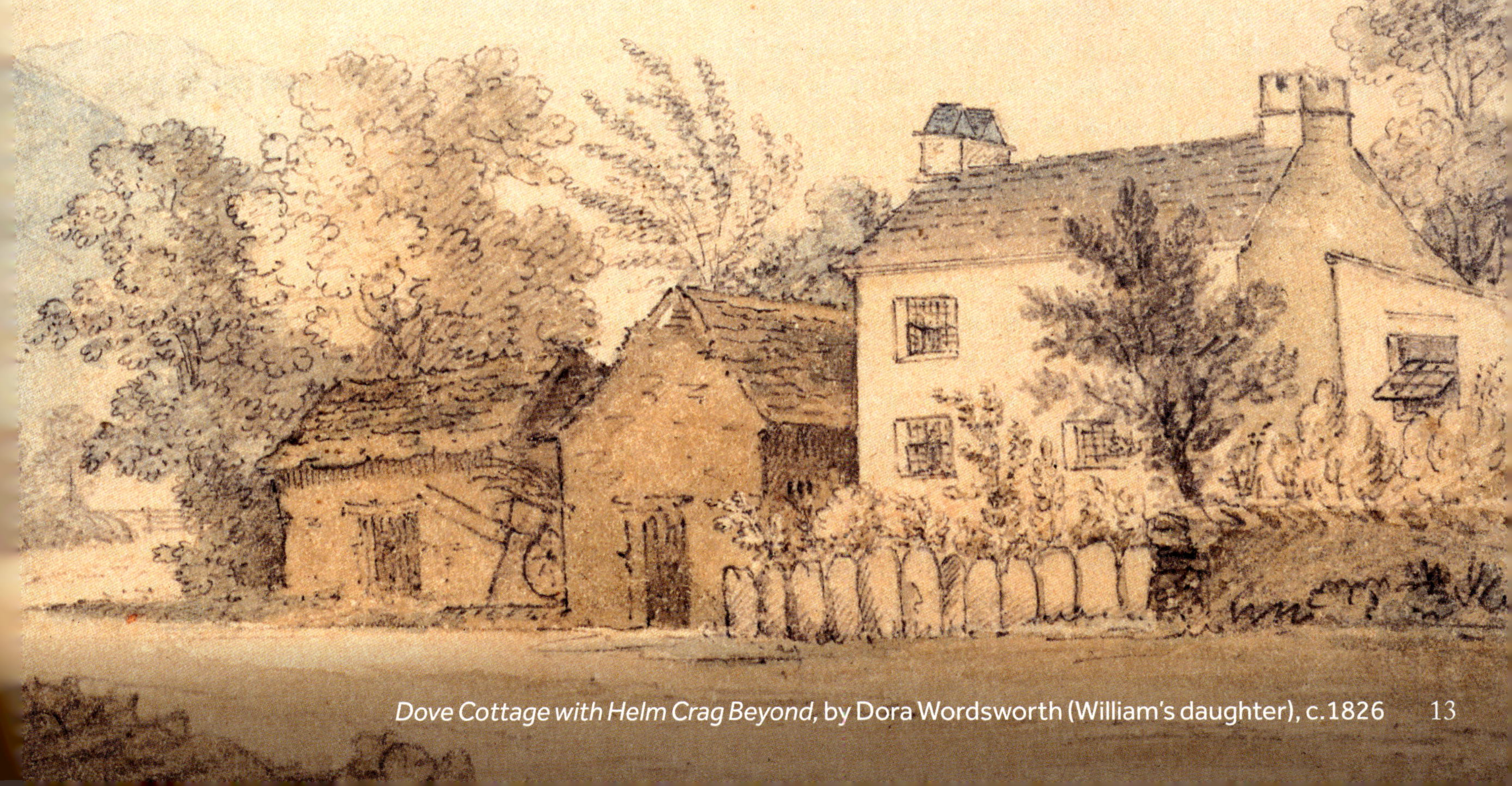

Dove Cottage with Helm Crag Beyond, by Dora Wordsworth (William's daughter), c.1826

Making themselves at home

Dorothy delighted in making the cottage comfortable. She spent her first Christmas in Grasmere sewing curtains, despite having dreadful toothache.

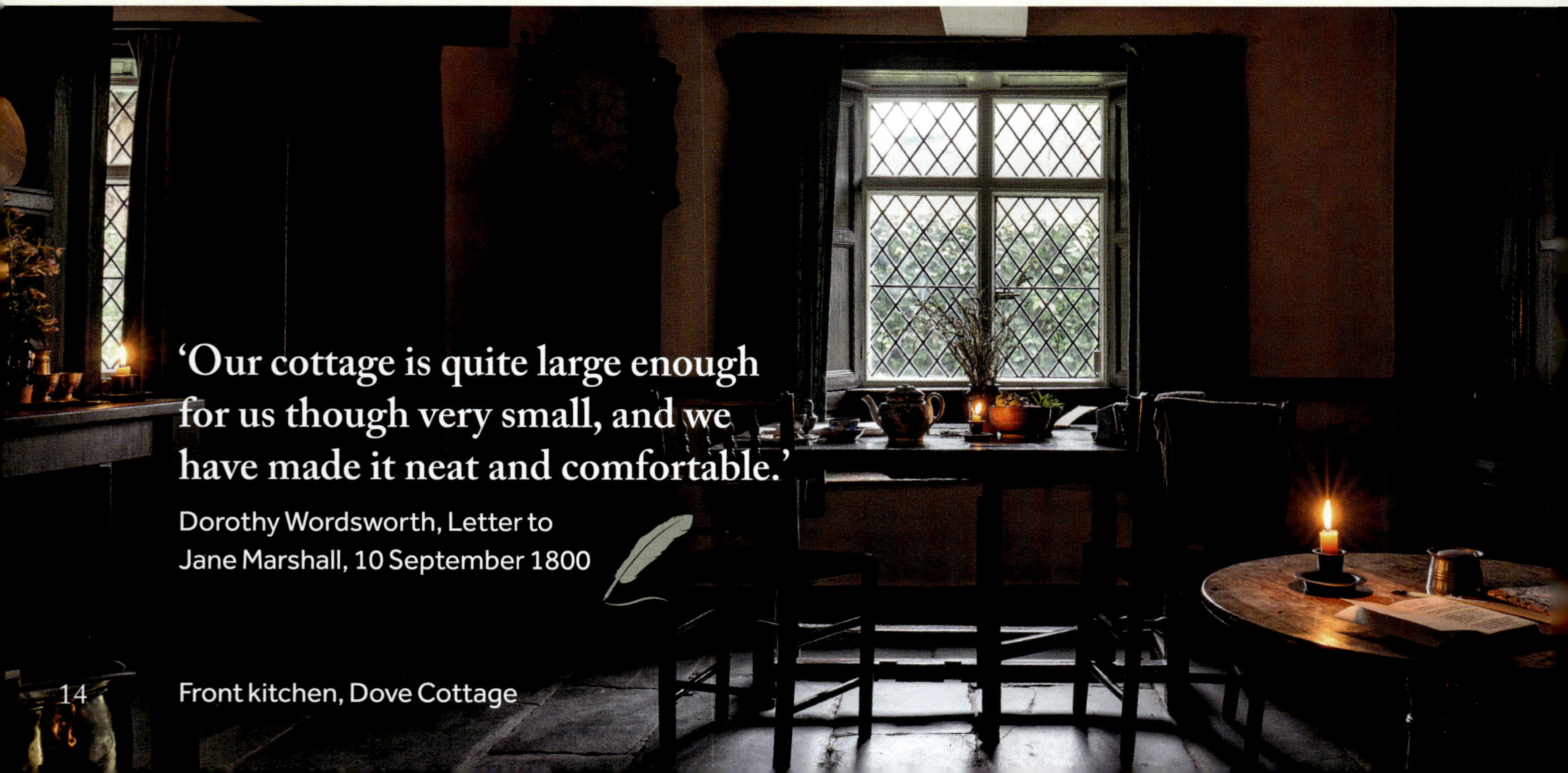

'Our cottage is quite large enough for us though very small, and we have made it neat and comfortable.'

Dorothy Wordsworth, Letter to Jane Marshall, 10 September 1800

Front kitchen, Dove Cottage

While William worked at his poems, Dorothy cooked and tidied and did most of the ironing and mending.

The Wordsworths employed one of their neighbours, Molly Fisher, to help with cleaning, lighting the fires, laundry and gardening. They had endless house guests, so there must have been a lot of washing.

This picture is by the Northumbrian artist Thomas Bewick, who lived around the same time as the Wordsworths.

What will the woman say when she turns round and sees what has happened to those nice clean shirts?

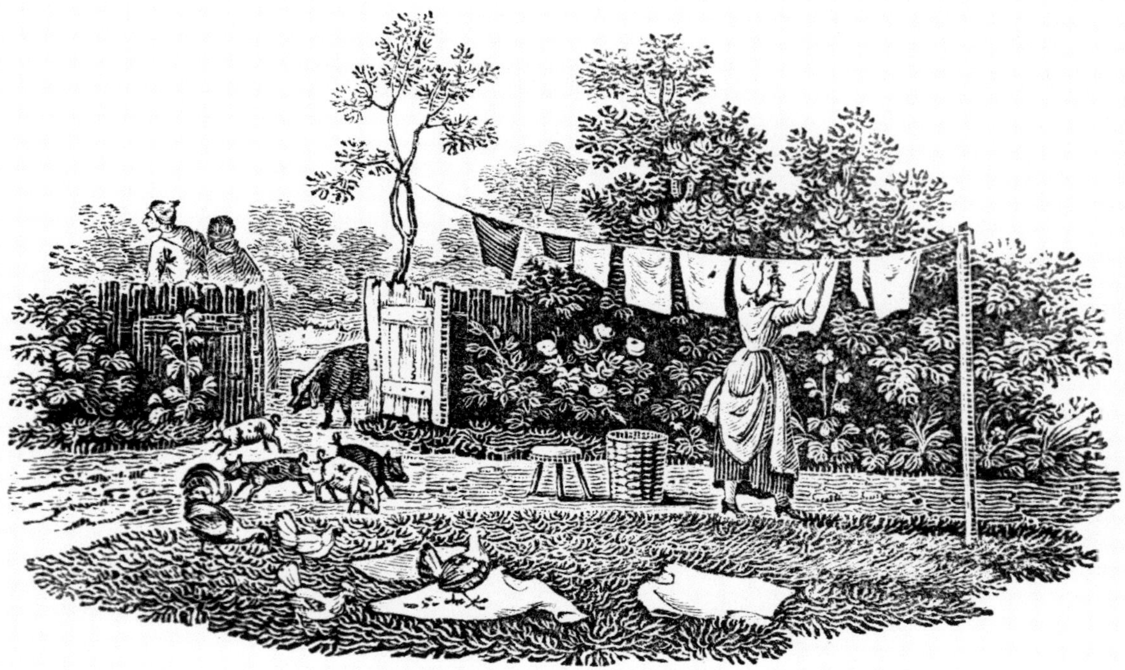

Reading and writing

Dorothy and William spent many hours reading – sometimes quietly, sometimes aloud, by themselves or with visiting friends.

On fine days they took their reading out of doors, to be immersed in nature. Other times, they sat cosily by the fire.

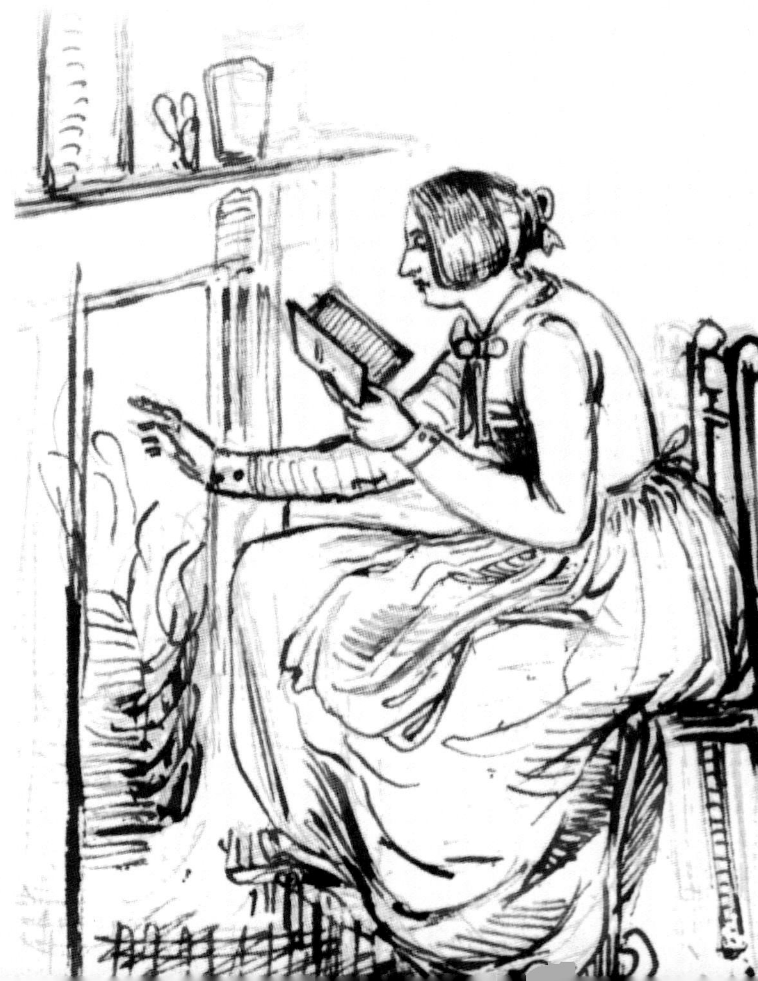

> ***This woman seems absorbed in her book, in spite of the cold!***
>
> *What do you suppose she is reading?*

Sketch by Mary Arnold, 1847

The Wordsworths read books of all kinds – history, literature, travel and poetry. Sometimes they copied their favourite passages into a 'Commonplace Book'.

In the upstairs sitting room of the little cottage they had a bookshelf; Dorothy was in charge of keeping the books in order.

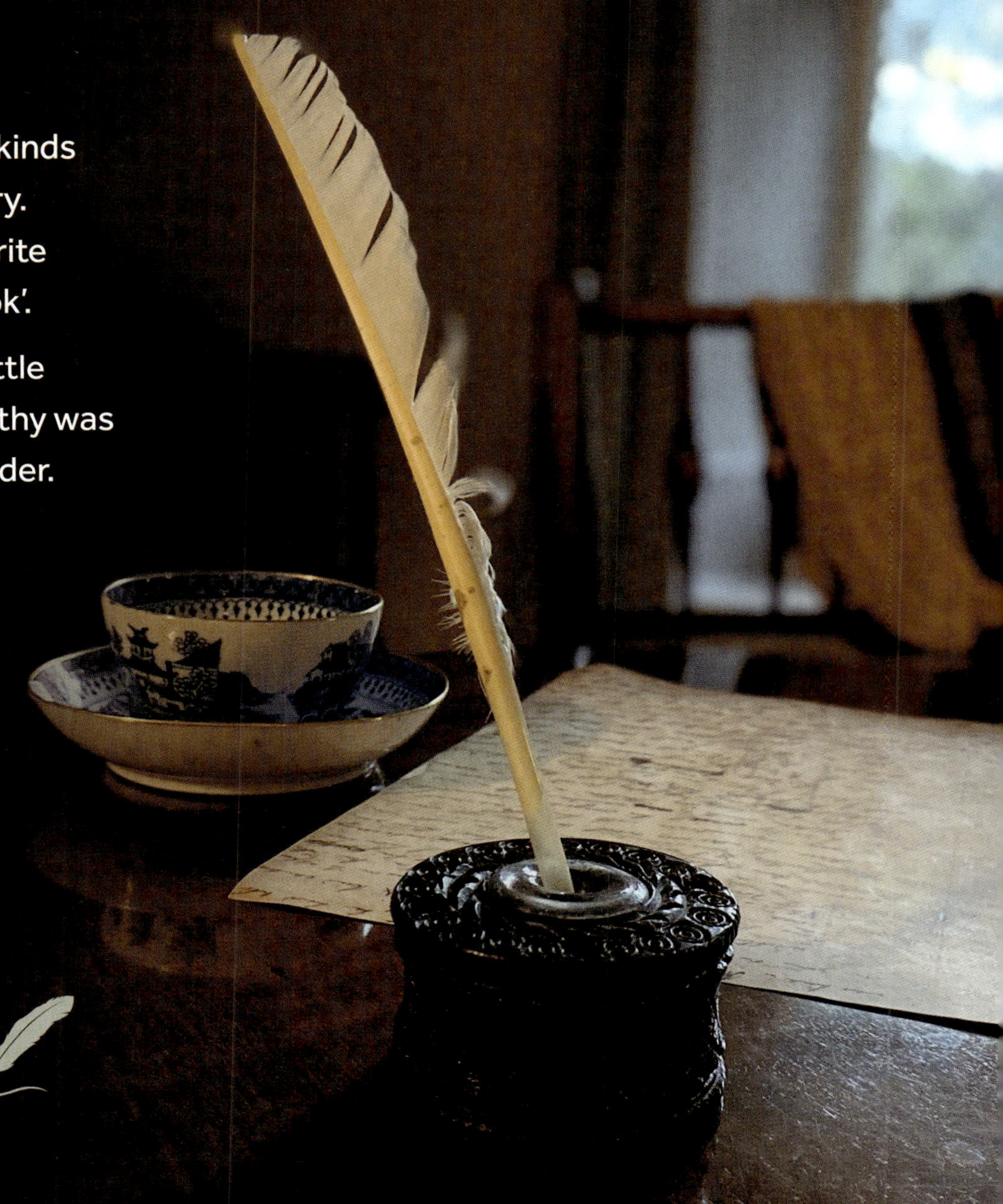

'Baked bread and giblet pie put books in order.'

Dorothy Wordsworth, *Grasmere Journals*, Wednesday 11 November 1801

Writing table in the upstairs sitting room at Dove Cottage

Partners in poetry

Dorothy's support was essential for William to create his poetry. Her conversation, observations and ideas inspired him.

Dorothy walked back and forth with William as he composed out of doors. Back at the cottage, Dorothy transcribed the poems line by line, often suggesting alterations and improvements.

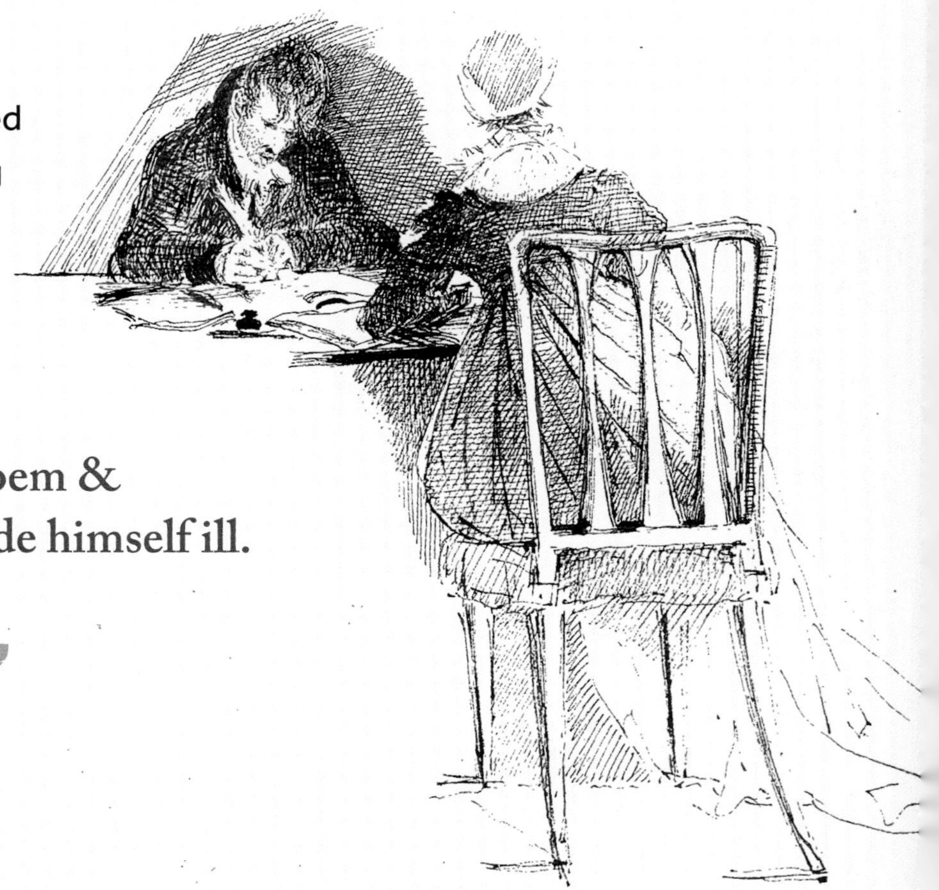

'William wrote out part of his poem & endeavoured to alter it, & so made himself ill. I copied out the rest for him.'

Dorothy Wordsworth, *Grasmere Journals,*
Tuesday 26 January 1802

Dorothy copied out thousands of lines of William's poetry. It was painstaking work.

It took seven years before William was happy with his long autobiographical poem 'The Pedlar'.

How do you suppose Dorothy felt when he kept changing his mind?

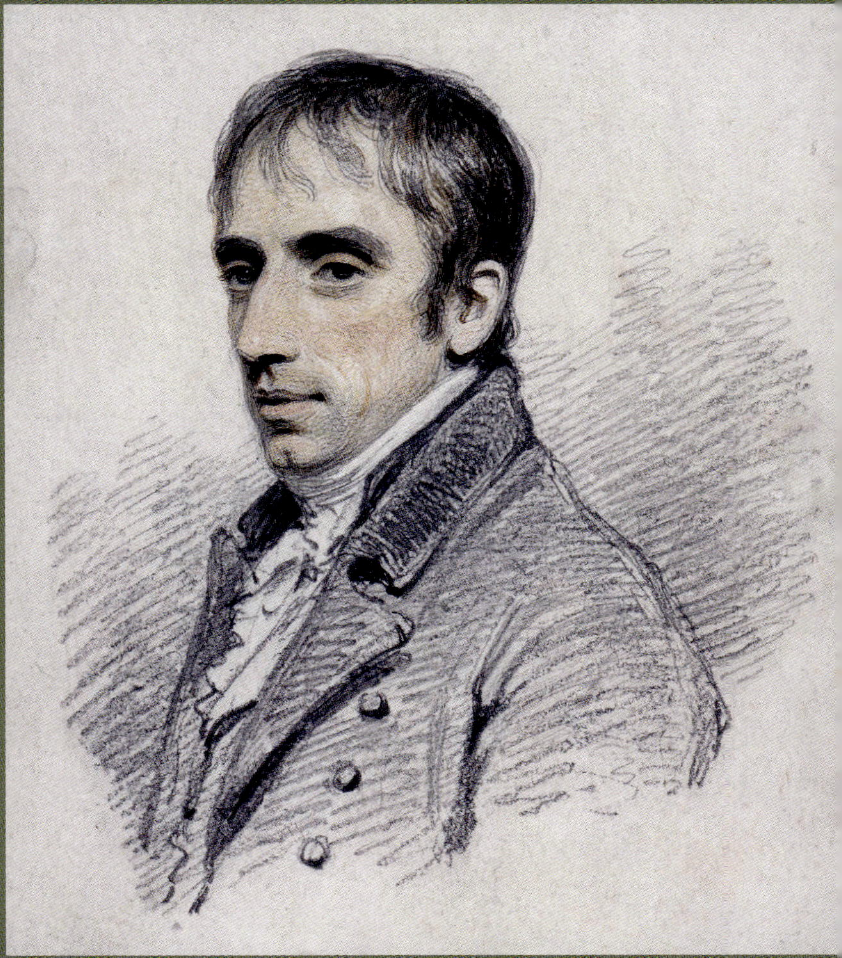

William Wordsworth, by Henry Edridge, 1806

'William left me at work altering some passages of the Pedlar & went into the orchard.'

Dorothy Wordsworth, *Grasmere Journals*, Sunday 14 February 1802

Dorothy's Grasmere Journals

On Wednesday 14 May 1800, Dorothy Wordsworth picked up a small, part-used, notebook and began to write about her day.

Dorothy kept up her journal for nearly three years. Some of her entries are several pages long, others just a few lines. If she was too busy to write, she would skip a day and catch up later.

When the first little notebook was full, Dorothy switched to another, then another.

'I resolved to write a journal & I set about keeping my resolve.'

Dorothy Wordsworth, *Grasmere Journals*, Wednesday 14 May 1800

If you kept a journal, what would you write about today?

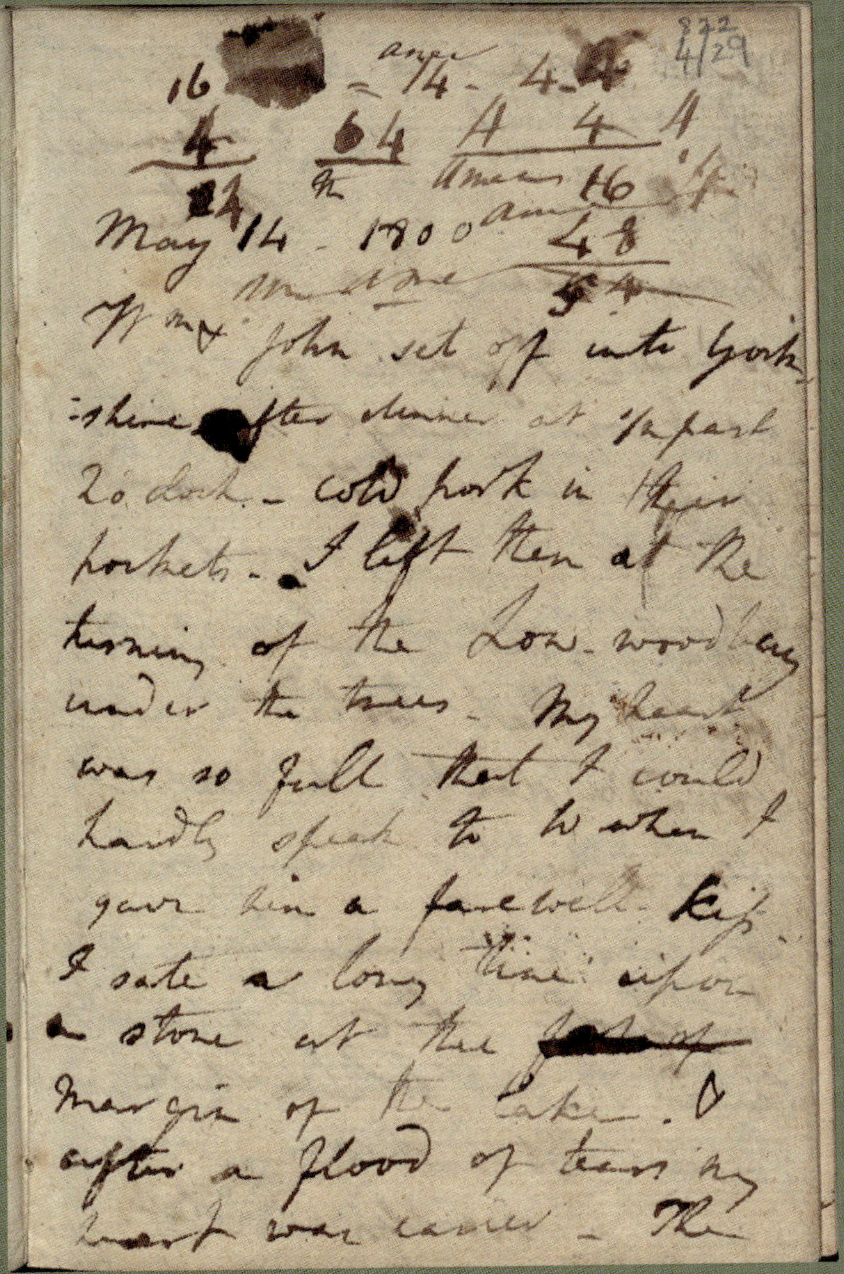

May 14 1800

Wm & John set off into Yorkshire after dinner at ½ past 2 o'clock – cold pork in their pockets. I left them at the turning of the Low-wood bay under the trees. My heart was so full that I could hardly speak to W when I gave him a farewell kiss. I sate a long time upon a stone at the margin of the lake & after a flood of tears my heart was easier. The

This is the first entry in Dorothy's journal, dated 14 May 1800. She didn't even start a fresh page!

Dorothy wrote her diary for William to read. Do you suppose he ever had difficulty deciphering her handwriting?

'Wm & John set off into Yorkshire after dinner at ½ past 2 o'clock – cold pork in their pockets.'

Dorothy Wordsworth, *Grasmere Journals*, Wednesday 14 May 1800

A journal of ordinary life

Most days, nothing out of the ordinary happened. Yet Dorothy Wordsworth found plenty to write about in her journal.

Dorothy wrote about doing the laundry, the cooking and the gardening; about going for walks – the flowers and trees she noticed, and the people she encountered. She wrote about the books she was reading and about helping William with his writing. She wrote about headaches and toothache; and, of course, she wrote about the weather.

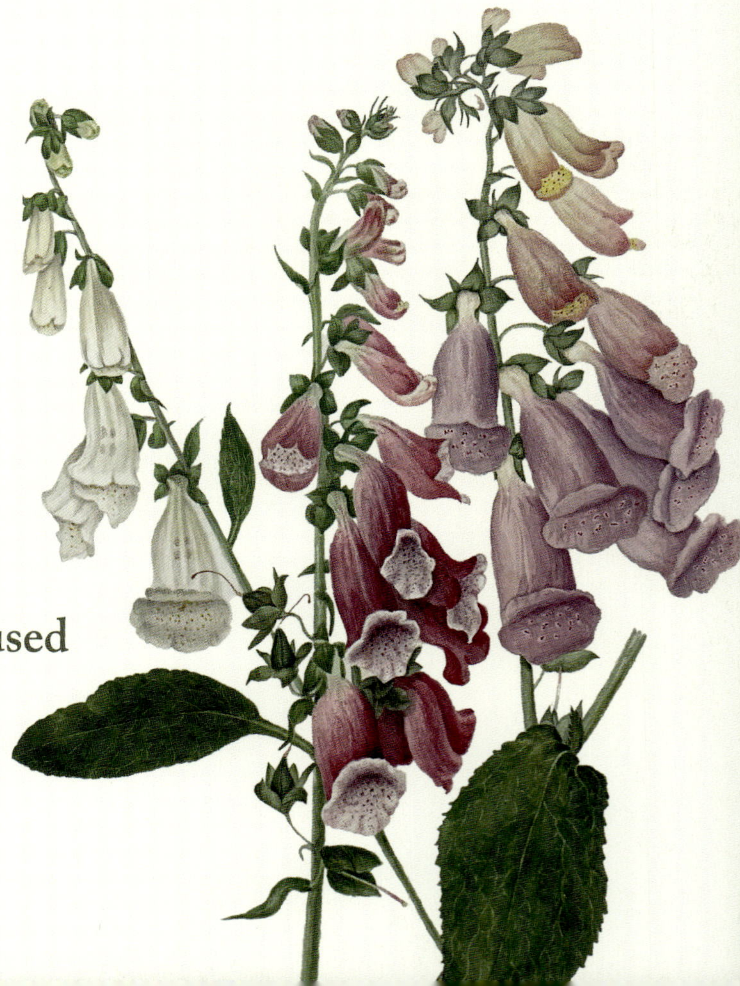

'Foxgloves very tall – with their heads budding. I went forward round the lake – I was much amused with the business of a pair of stone chats.'

Dorothy Wordsworth, *Grasmere Journals,*
Friday 16 May 1800

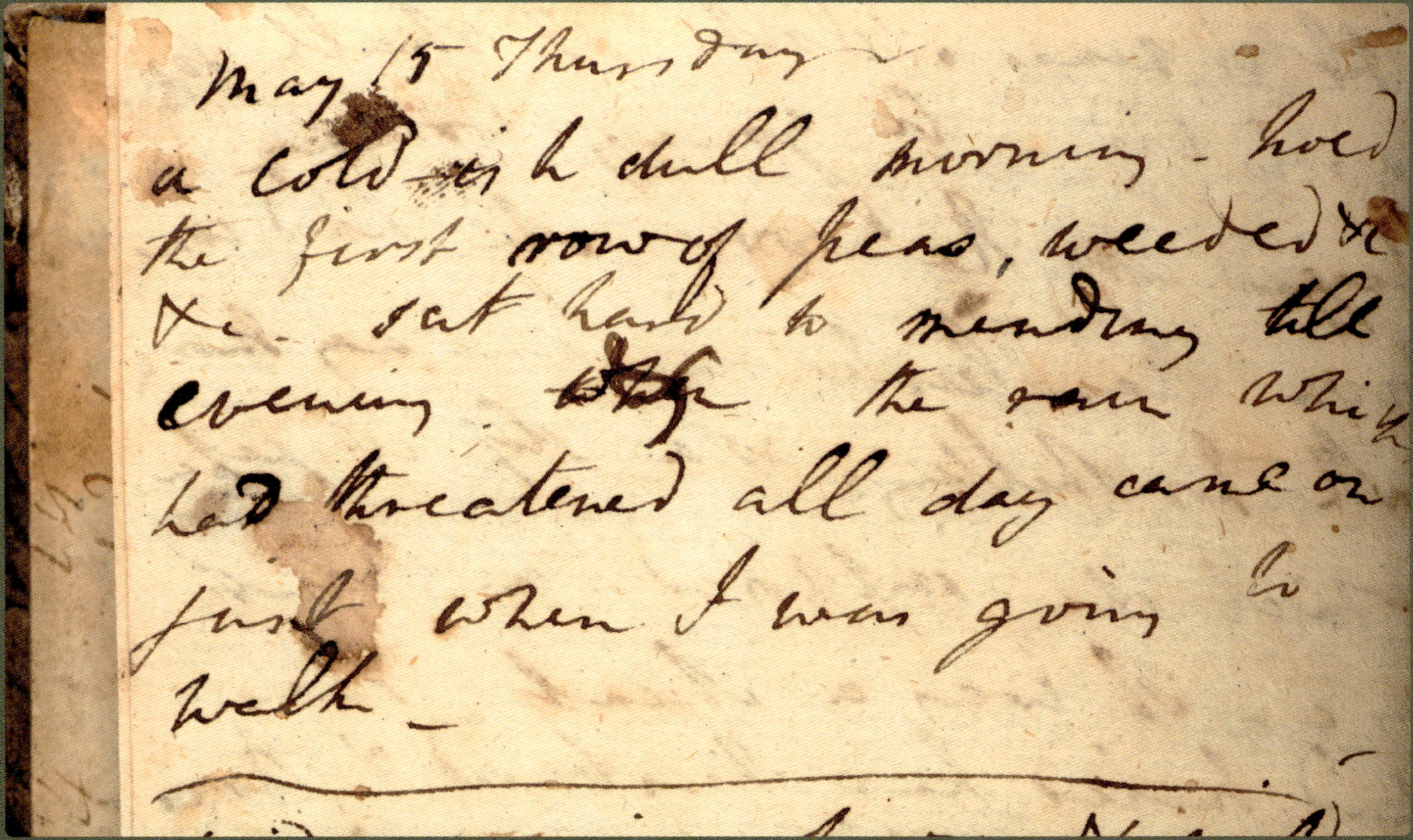
May 15 Thursday
a coldish dull morning - hoed
the first row of peas, weeded &c
&c - sat hard to mending till
evening the rain which
had threatened all day came on
just when I was going to
walk -

'May 15 Thursday

A coldish dull morning – hoed the first row of peas, weeded &c &c – sat hard to mending till evening. The rain which had threatened all day came on just when I was going to walk –'

Dorothy Wordsworth, *Grasmere Journals,*
Thursday 15 May 1800

Letters

As well as writing her journal and transcribing William's poems, Dorothy Wordsworth wrote hundreds of letters to friends and family.

Letters were very important to Dorothy. She wrote at length – often filling several large sheets – and was always disappointed on days when no letters came in return.

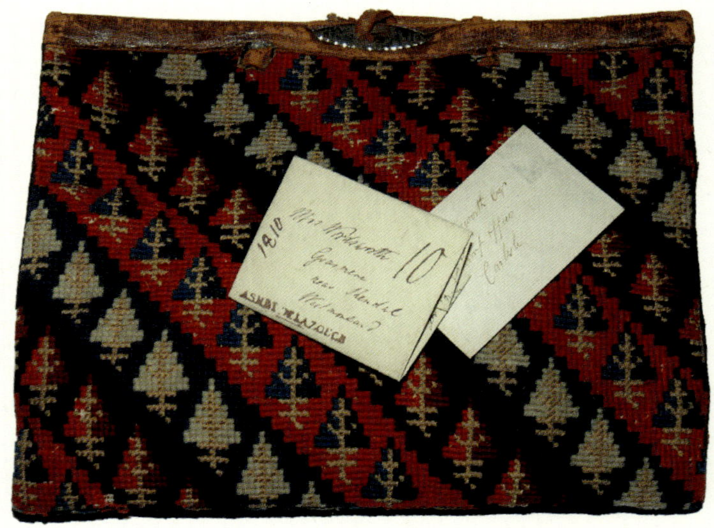

The Wordsworths used this colourful tapestry bag for carrying letters to and from the post office. Dorothy often walked as far as Ambleside (three miles each way) to deliver and collect letters.

'No letters. No papers. It was a very cold cheerless evening.'

Dorothy Wordsworth, *Grasmere Journal,* Tuesday 10 June 1800

Pens and ink

The Wordsworths required a constant supply of pens and ink.

Pens were handmade from feathers, trimmed down with a sharp penknife. The point of the quill was shaped to form a nib, with a tiny slit in the end to hold the ink.

Ink could be made at home too, but it took three days to prepare, so it was best not to run out.

To make ink

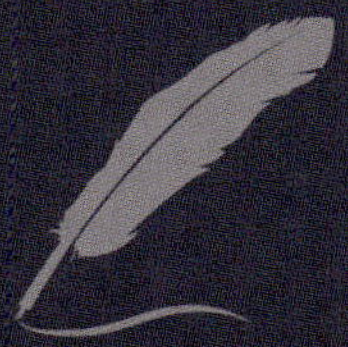

1oz gum arabic
3oz oak galls
1oz sulphate of iron
A quart of warm water

Put as much water upon the gum as will dissolve it and the rest on the galls & iron. Let it stand three days without a cork – shake it – after three days add the gum & it is fit for use.

Recipe from the Wordsworths' Commonplace Book

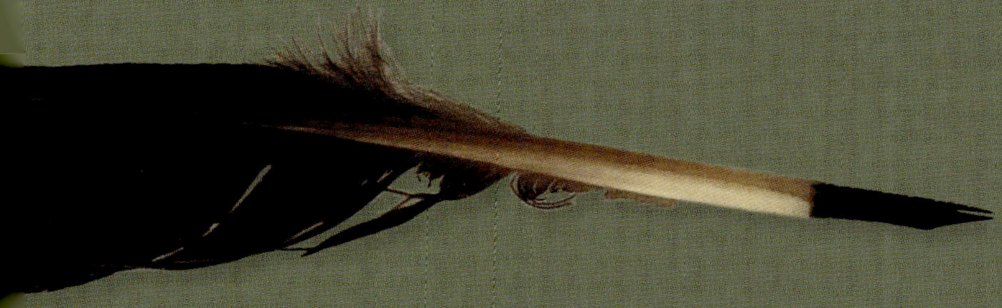

This quill pen once belonged to Sara Hutchinson, Dorothy's sister-in-law.

What would your handwriting be like if you used a quill pen?

Outside the window

In the Spring of 1802, Dorothy watched, fascinated, as a pair of swallows built their nest outside her bedroom window.

A week later, the near-complete nest suddenly collapsed onto the window ledge. Dorothy was almost as distressed as the birds themselves.

Undeterred, the swallows quickly set about the task of rebuilding. On Tuesday 5 July, Dorothy was pleased to record:
'The swallows have completed their beautiful nest. I baked bread and pies.'

It has been suggested that the birds which Dorothy described as swallows were in fact house martins – an easy mistake to make!

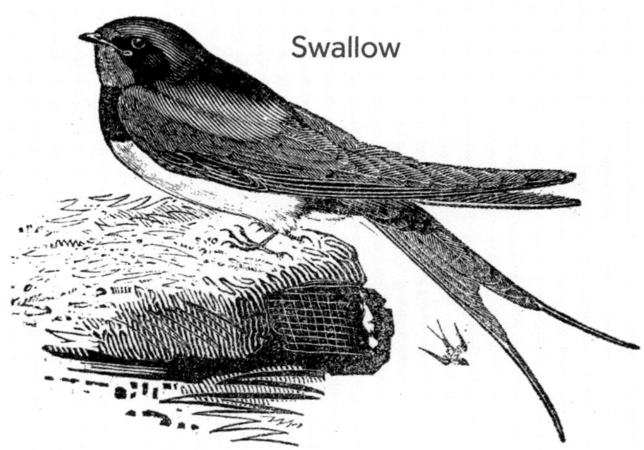

Swallow

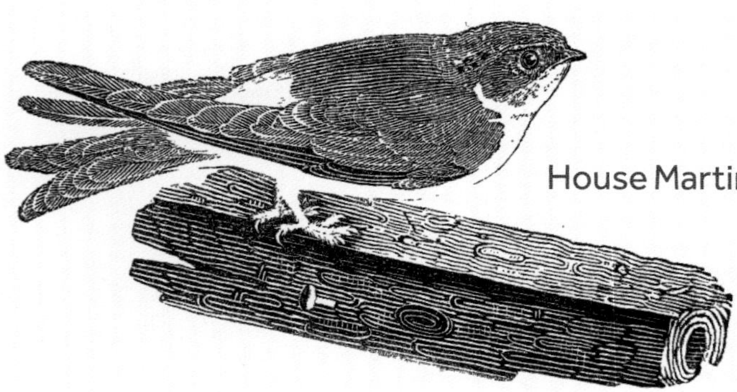

House Martin

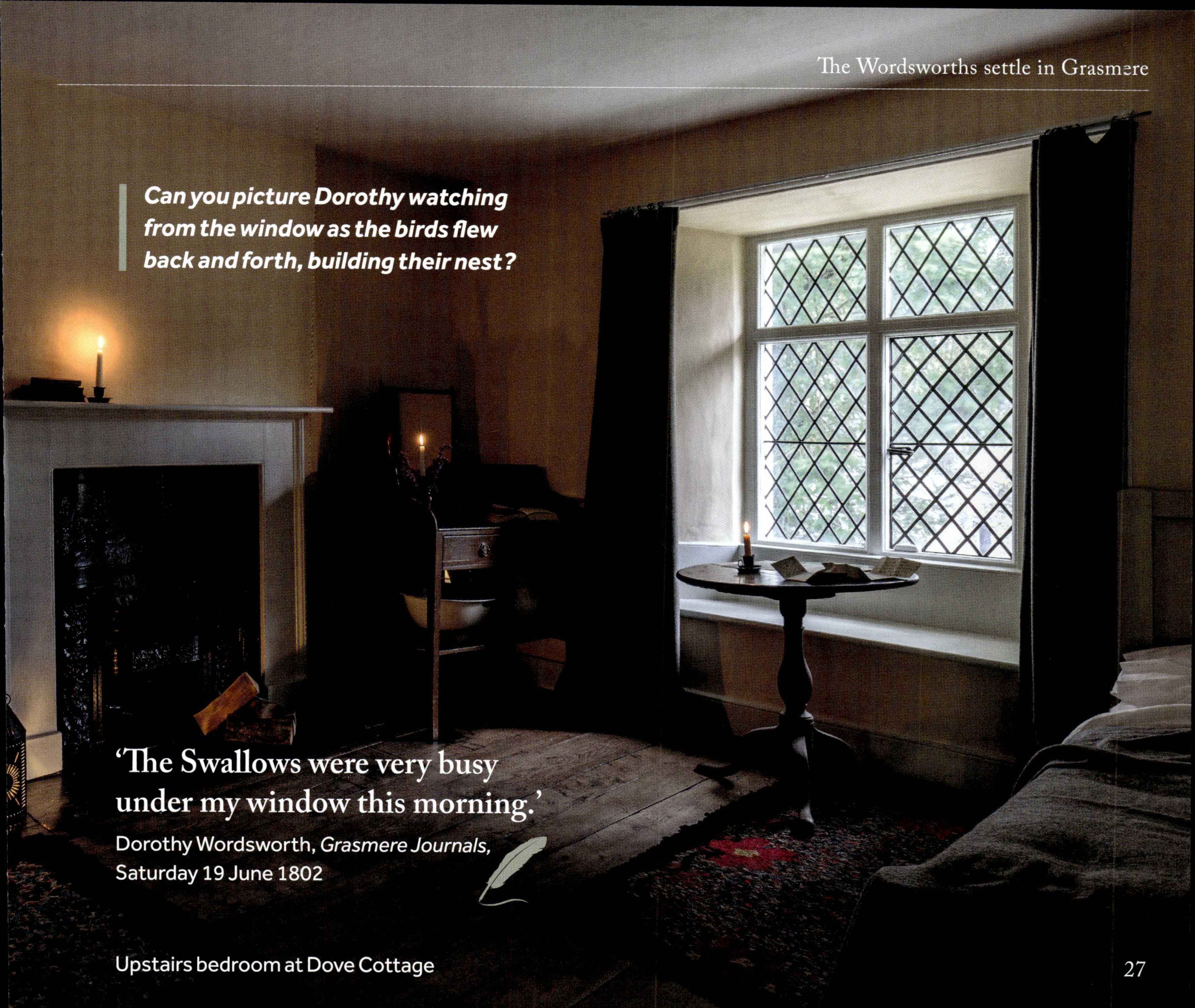

Can you picture Dorothy watching from the window as the birds flew back and forth, building their nest?

'The Swallows were very busy under my window this morning.'

Dorothy Wordsworth, *Grasmere Journals*, Saturday 19 June 1802

Upstairs bedroom at Dove Cottage

In the garden

Dorothy was proud of the little garden that she and William created around the cottage. They had space to grow flowers and vegetables and to keep bees in hives against the wall.

Sometimes the weather got the better of them. On Monday 5 July 1802, after a period of heavy rain, Dorothy wrote in her journal: *'The Roses in the garden are fretted & battered & quite spoiled. The honeysuckle though in its glory is sadly teazed. The peas are beaten down. The Scarlet Beans want sticking. The garden is overrun with weeds.'*

'I shelled peas, gathered beans, & worked in the garden till ½ past 12.'

Dorothy Wordsworth, *Grasmere Journals*,
Saturday 23 August 1800

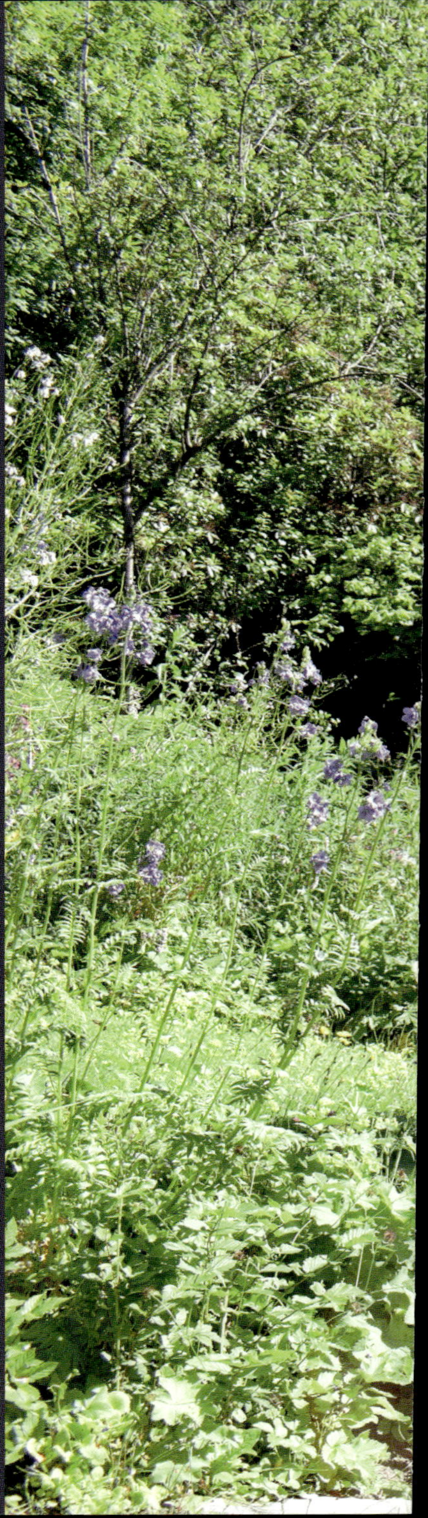

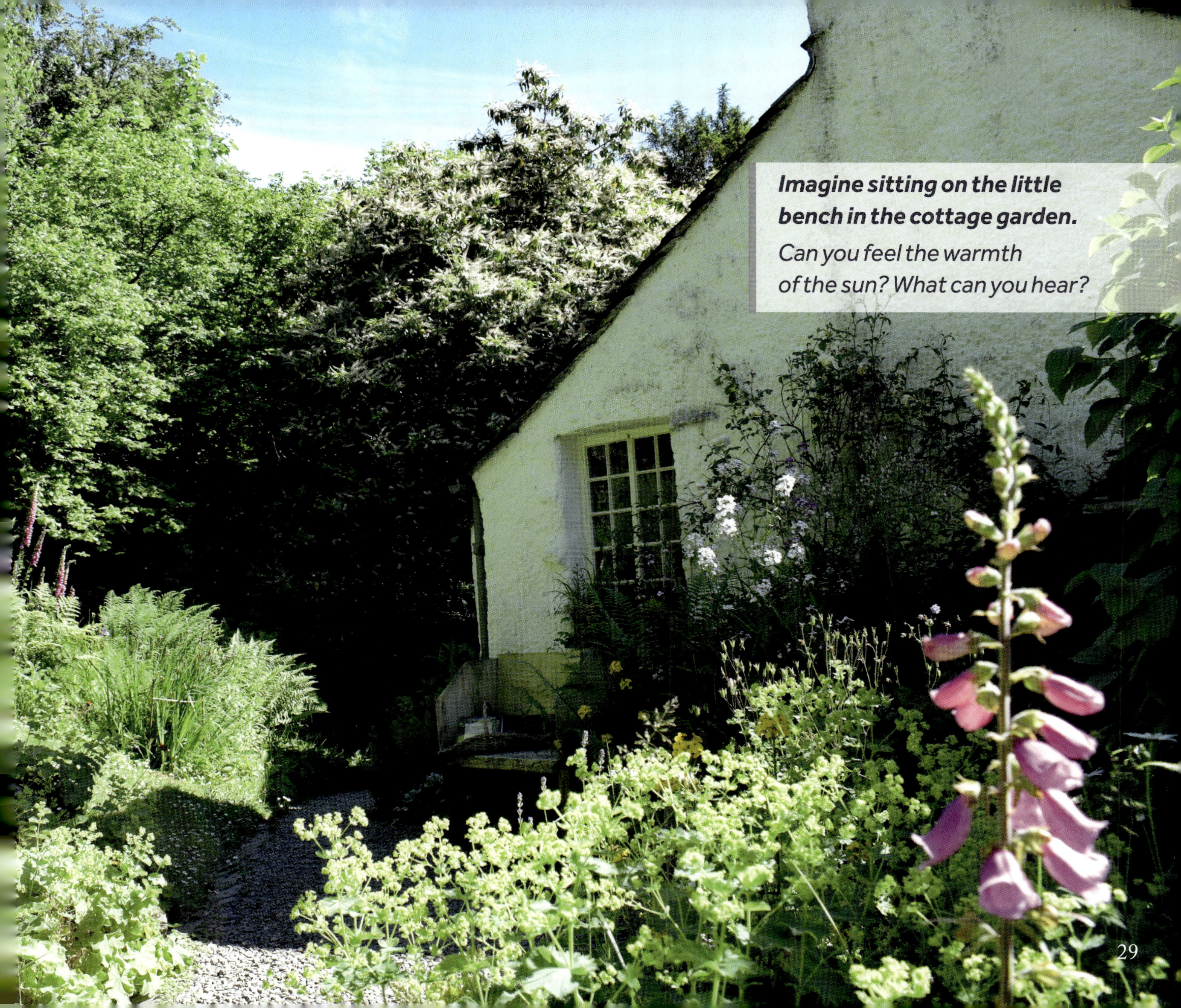

Imagine sitting on the little bench in the cottage garden.

Can you feel the warmth of the sun? What can you hear?

A sweet morning in the orchard

The steeply sloping orchard at the back of the house was more secluded than the garden at the front. Perfect for reading, drinking tea, composing poetry and resting under the trees.

On 6 May 1802 Dorothy took her journal into the orchard, sat down under the trees, and recorded everything she could hear and see. What a wonderful thing to do on a fine spring morning!

Thrush

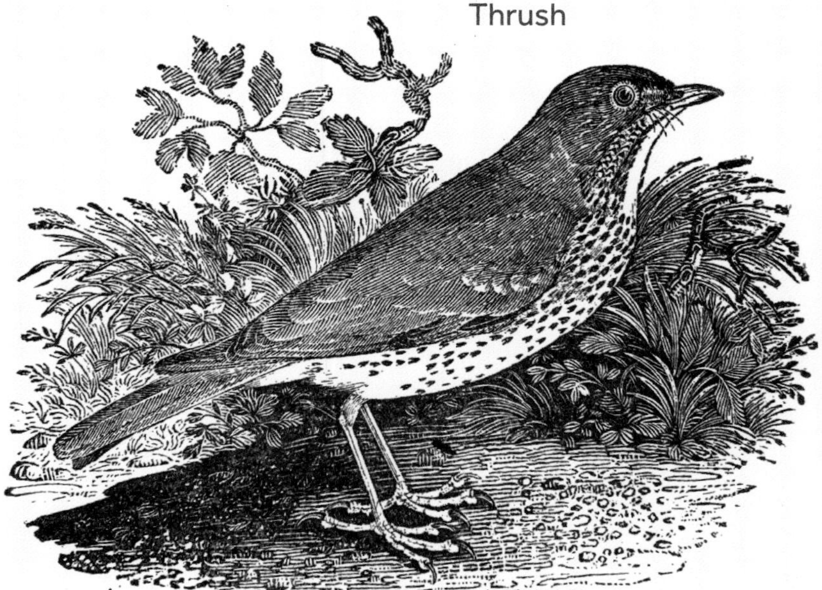

'The Throstle [thrush] is distinguished among our singing birds by the clearness and fullness of its note.'

Thomas Bewick, *History of British Birds*, 1797

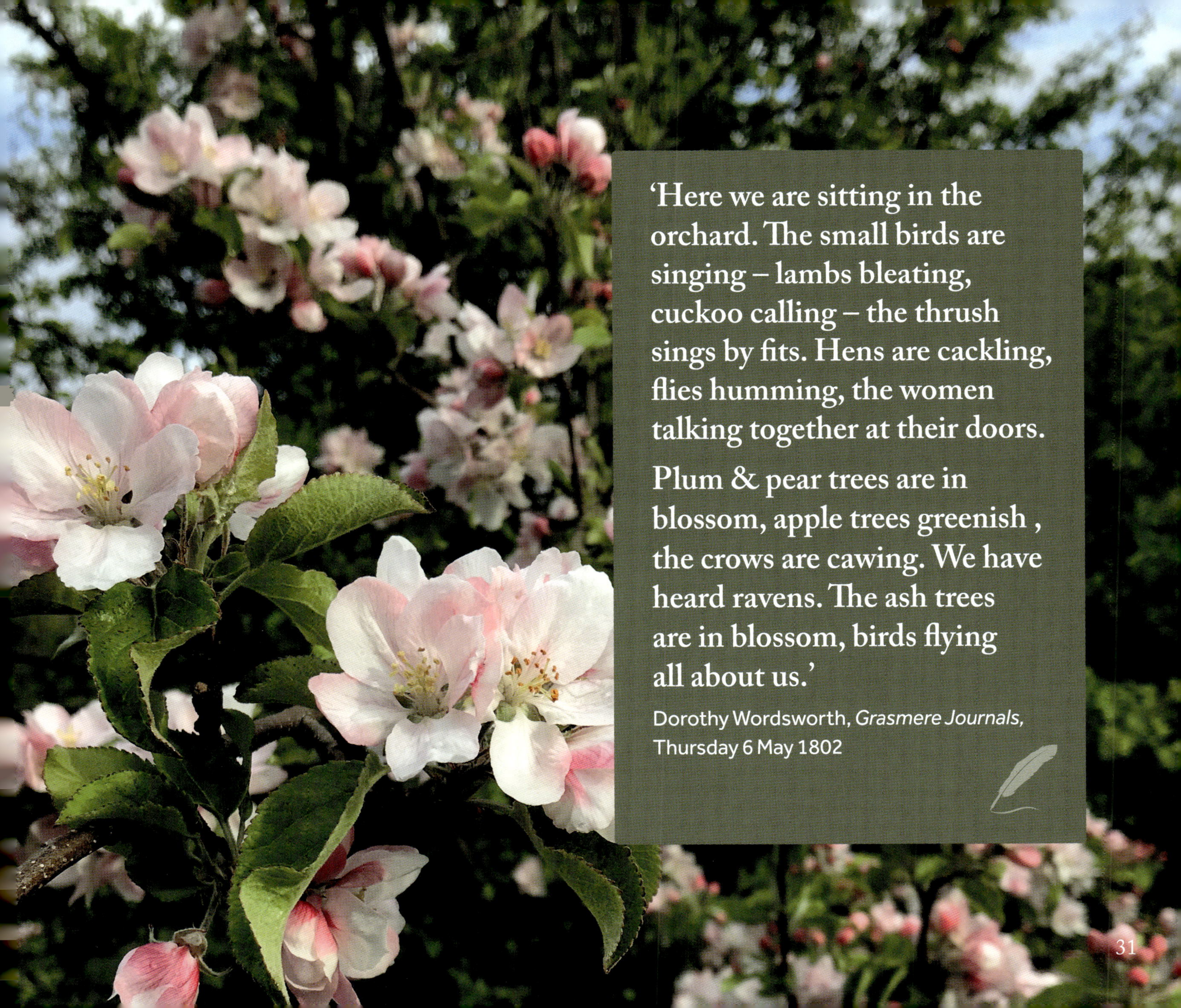

‘Here we are sitting in the orchard. The small birds are singing – lambs bleating, cuckoo calling – the thrush sings by fits. Hens are cackling, flies humming, the women talking together at their doors.

Plum & pear trees are in blossom, apple trees greenish , the crows are cawing. We have heard ravens. The ash trees are in blossom, birds flying all about us.’

Dorothy Wordsworth, *Grasmere Journals*, Thursday 6 May 1802

A pioneer on the hills

Dorothy was a keen and vigorous walker. From the cottage, she could walk easily round Grasmere Lake and Rydal Water. For a longer stretch she could climb Loughrigg Fell or take the path into Easedale.

Dorothy also relished more adventurous expeditions. In October 1818, she and her friend Mary Barker made an ascent of Scafell Pike – England's highest mountain.

Afterwards, Dorothy wrote a remarkable description of the climb – the earliest-known such account to be written by a woman.

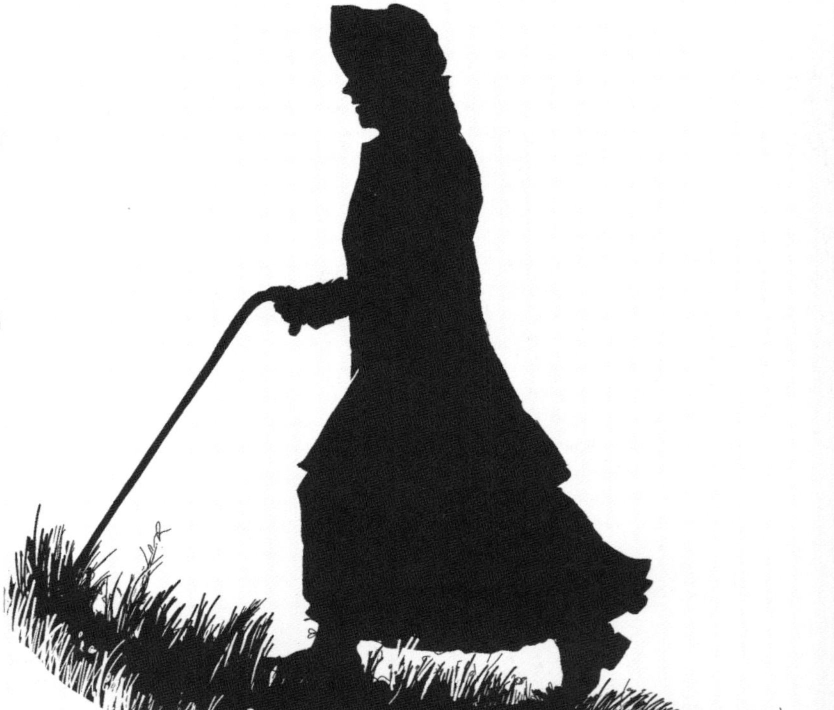

'The majesty of the mountains below and close to us, is not to be conceived.'

Dorothy Wordsworth, Letter to William Johnson, 21 October 1818

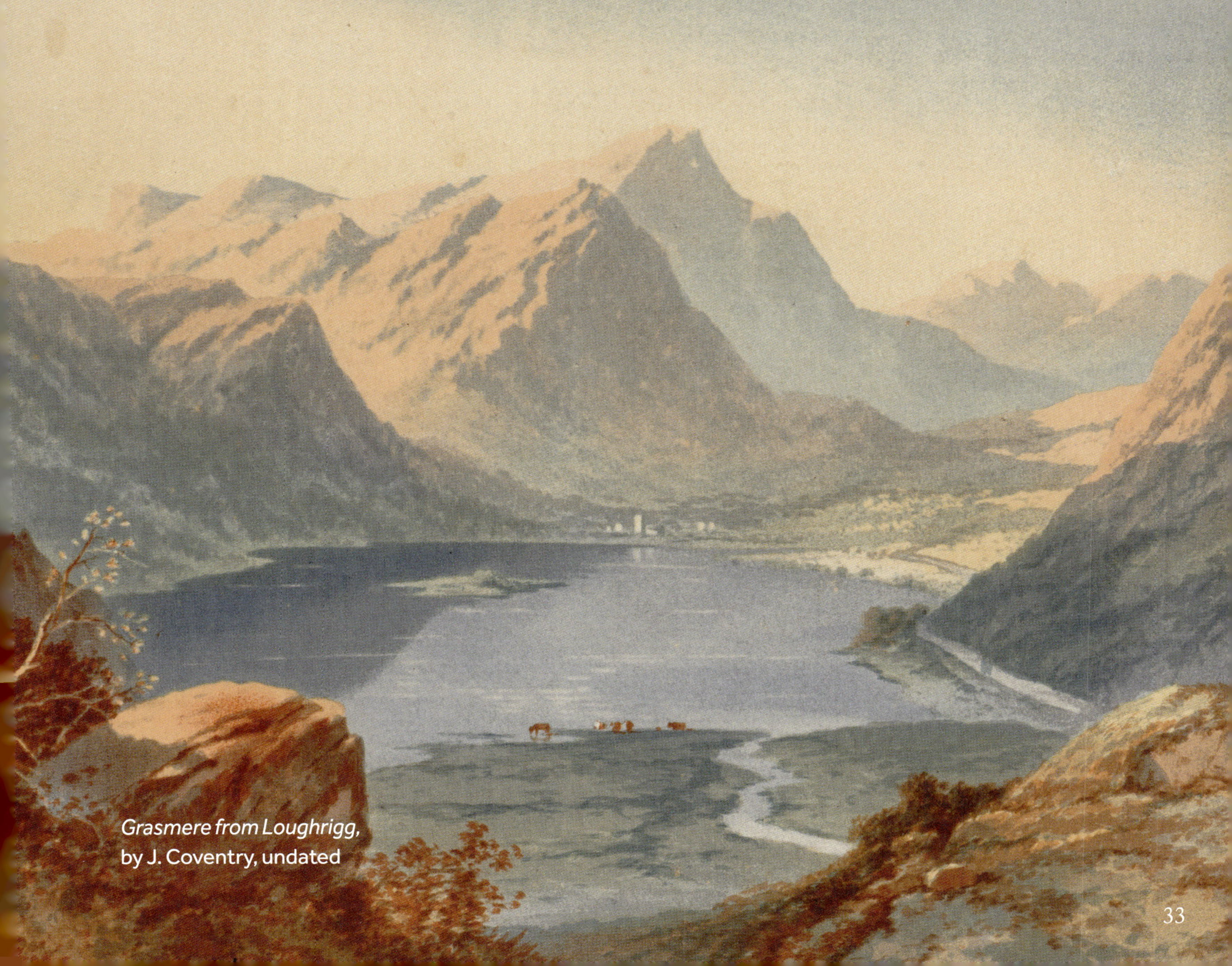

Grasmere from Loughrigg,
by J. Coventry, undated

Going fishing

Dorothy recorded several fishing expeditions during the summer of 1800, while her younger brother John Wordsworth was visiting.

On 11 June 1800 William and John brought home two pikes, which they ate for dinner the next day. They went out on the lake again two days later and caught another pike weighing seven and a half pounds.

'We went on the lake to set pike floats … returned to dinner, two pikes boiled and roasted.'

Dorothy Wordsworth, *Grasmere Journals.* 11 June 1800

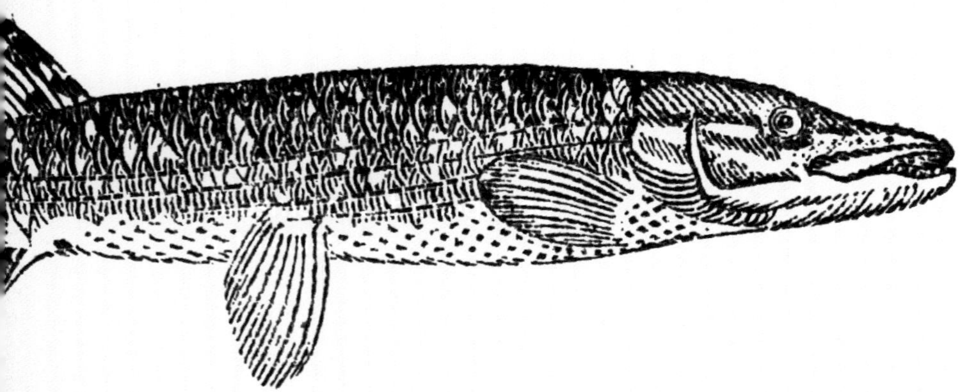

What must Dorothy have thought when she had to keep on cooking pike for dinner?

‘Grasmere Lake a beautiful image of stillness, clear as glass, reflecting all things.’

Dorothy Wordsworth, *Grasmere Journals*, Saturday 26 December 1801

Grasmere with Loughrigg in the distance, by William Green, 1802

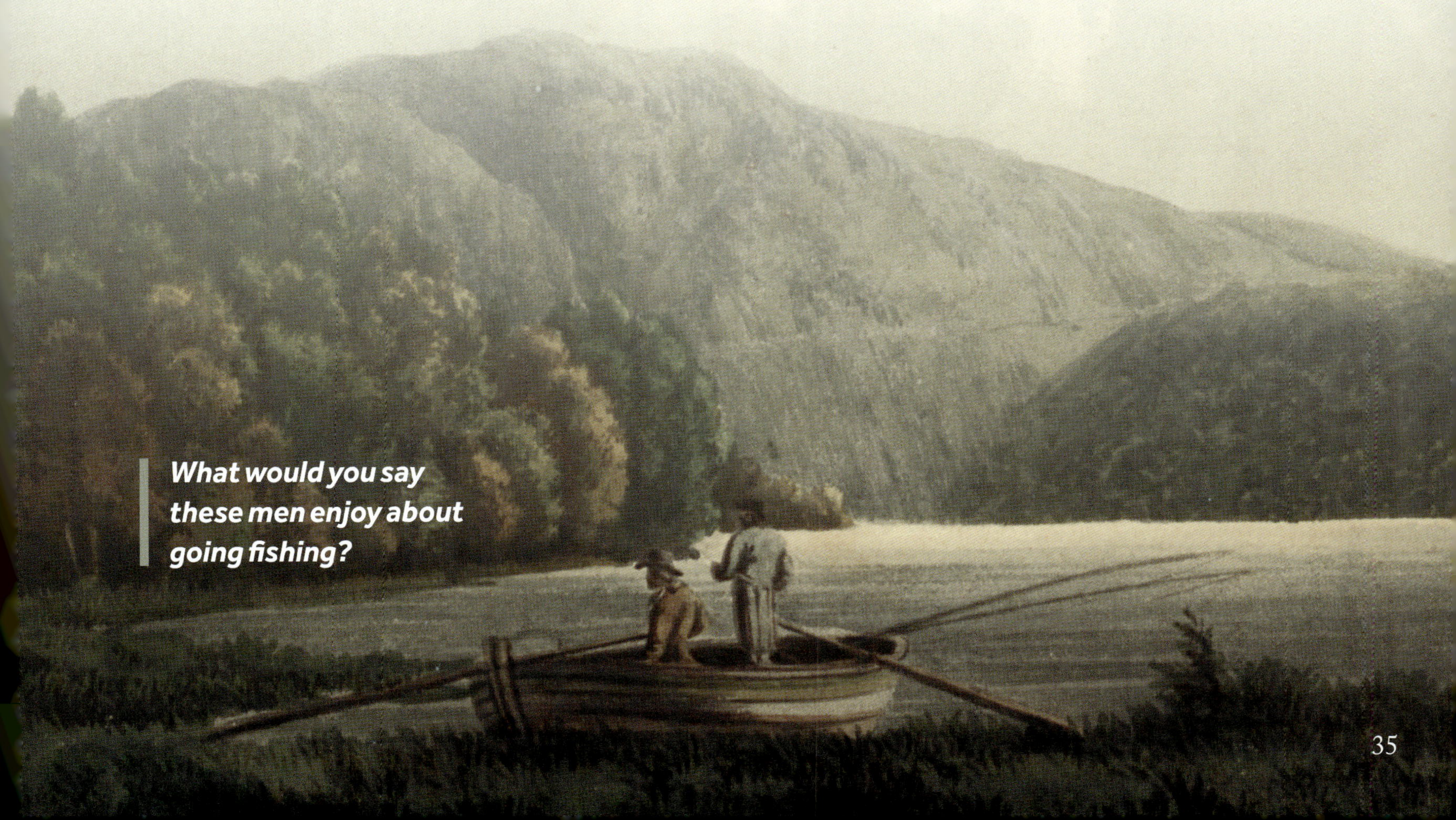

What would you say these men enjoy about going fishing?

Night-time walking

Dorothy and William often walked at night – to visit friends, deliver letters, or for the sheer pleasure of being out and about under the moon and stars.

On mild nights they saw glowworms. When it was fine, the moon rising above the fell appeared startlingly beautiful.

On wild and windy nights, the hurrying clouds lent added drama to the scene.

In winter, the roads were cold and slippery, but it was worth going out to catch a glimpse of the snow-covered mountains in the moonlight.

'A very fine moonlight night – The moonshine like herrings in the water.'

Dorothy Wordsworth, *Grasmere Journals*, Friday 31 October 1800

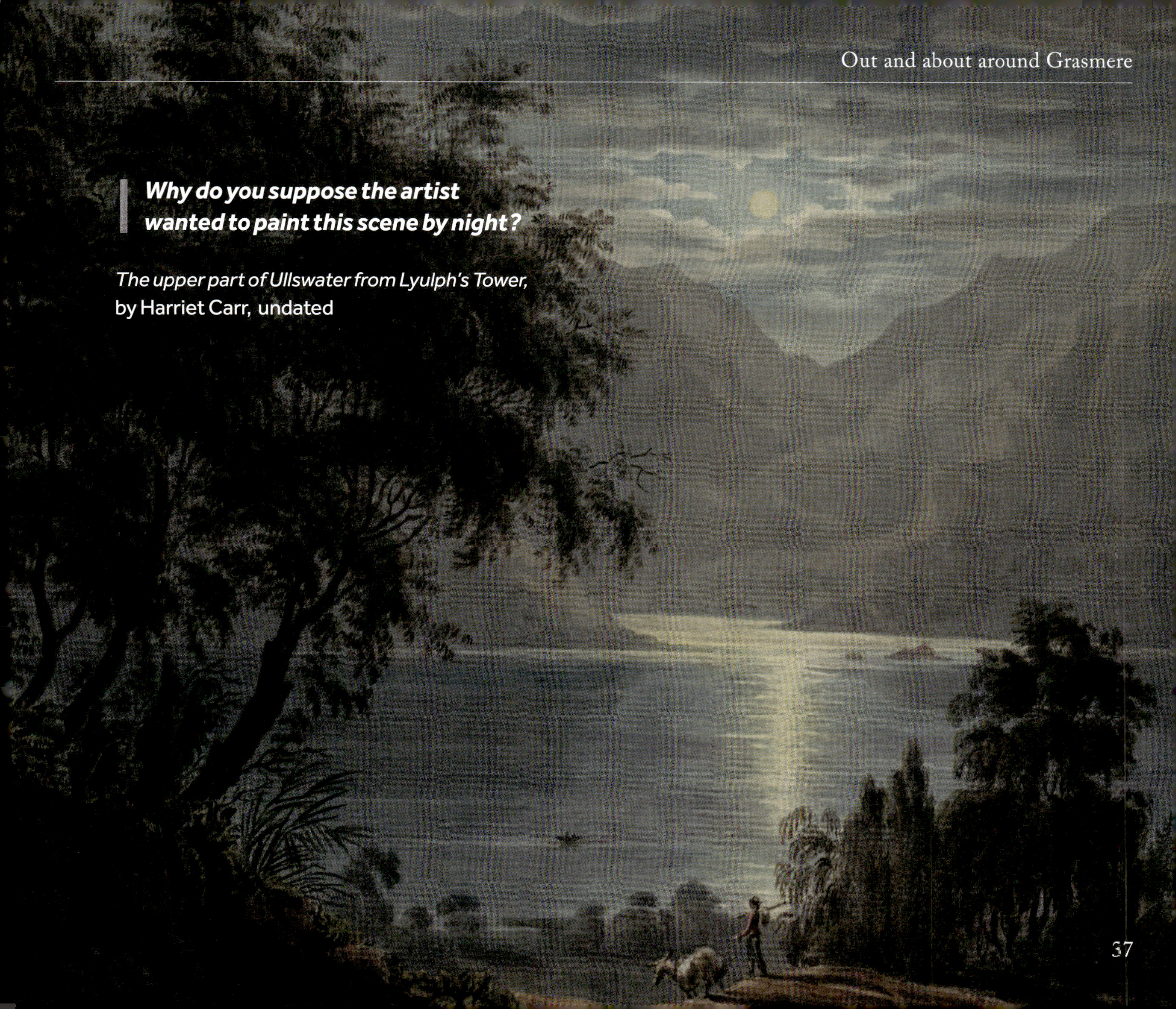

Why do you suppose the artist wanted to paint this scene by night?

The upper part of Ullswater from Lyulph's Tower,
by Harriet Carr, undated

Daffodils

On Thursday 15 April 1802, Dorothy and William were out walking near Ullswater. There was a furious wind and the lake was rough. They were almost tempted to give up, but were encouraged by the sight of primroses and violets by the roadside.

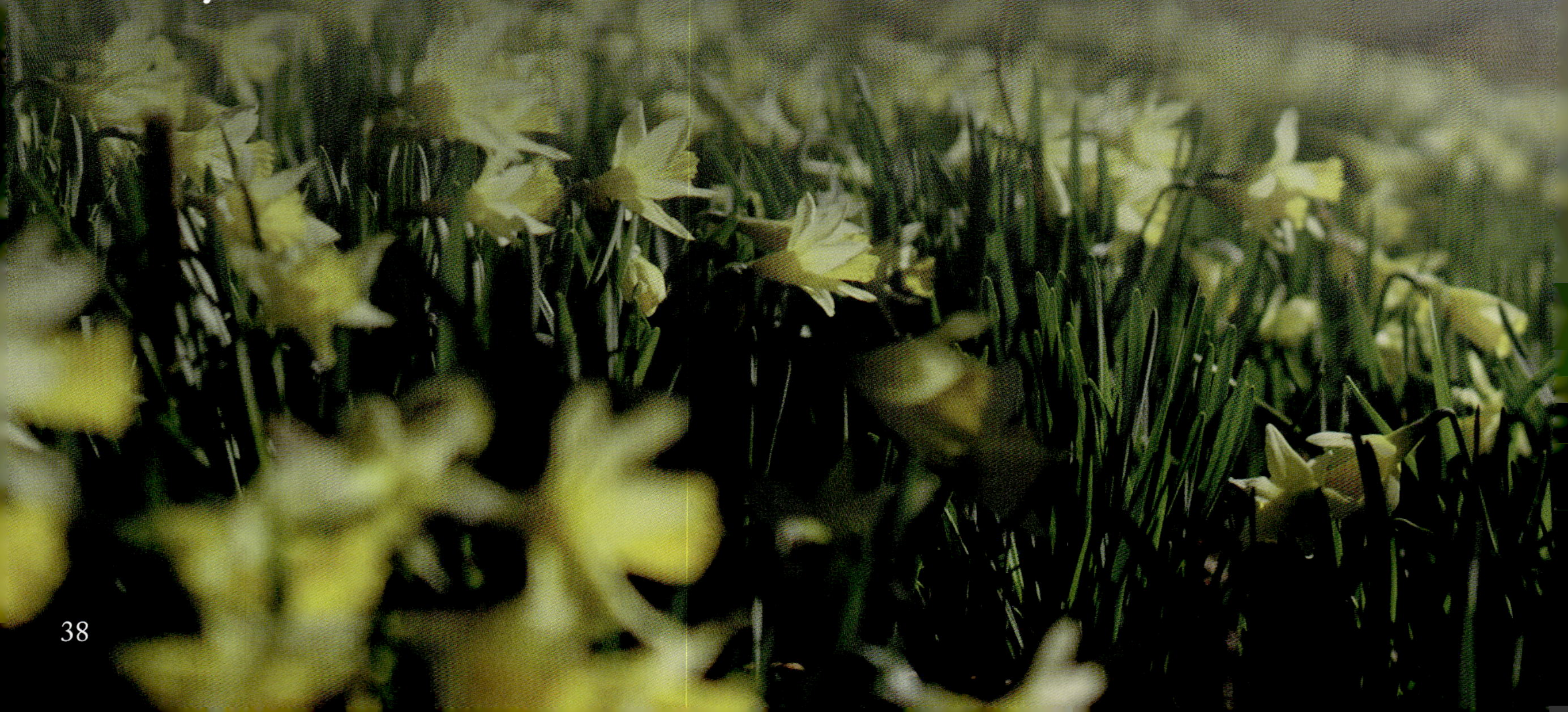

As they walked through the woods, they saw the daffodils – at first a few, then more and more – tossing, reeling and dancing in the wind.

Imagine if William and Dorothy had been deterred by the wind and had never seen the daffodils!

'I never saw daffodils so beautiful. They grew among the mossy stones about and about them, some rested their heads upon these stones as on a pillow for weariness and the rest tossed and reeled and danced and seemed as if they verily laughed with the wind that blew upon them over the lake, they looked so gay ever glancing ever changing.'

Dorothy Wordsworth, *Grasmere Journals*, Thursday 15 April 1802

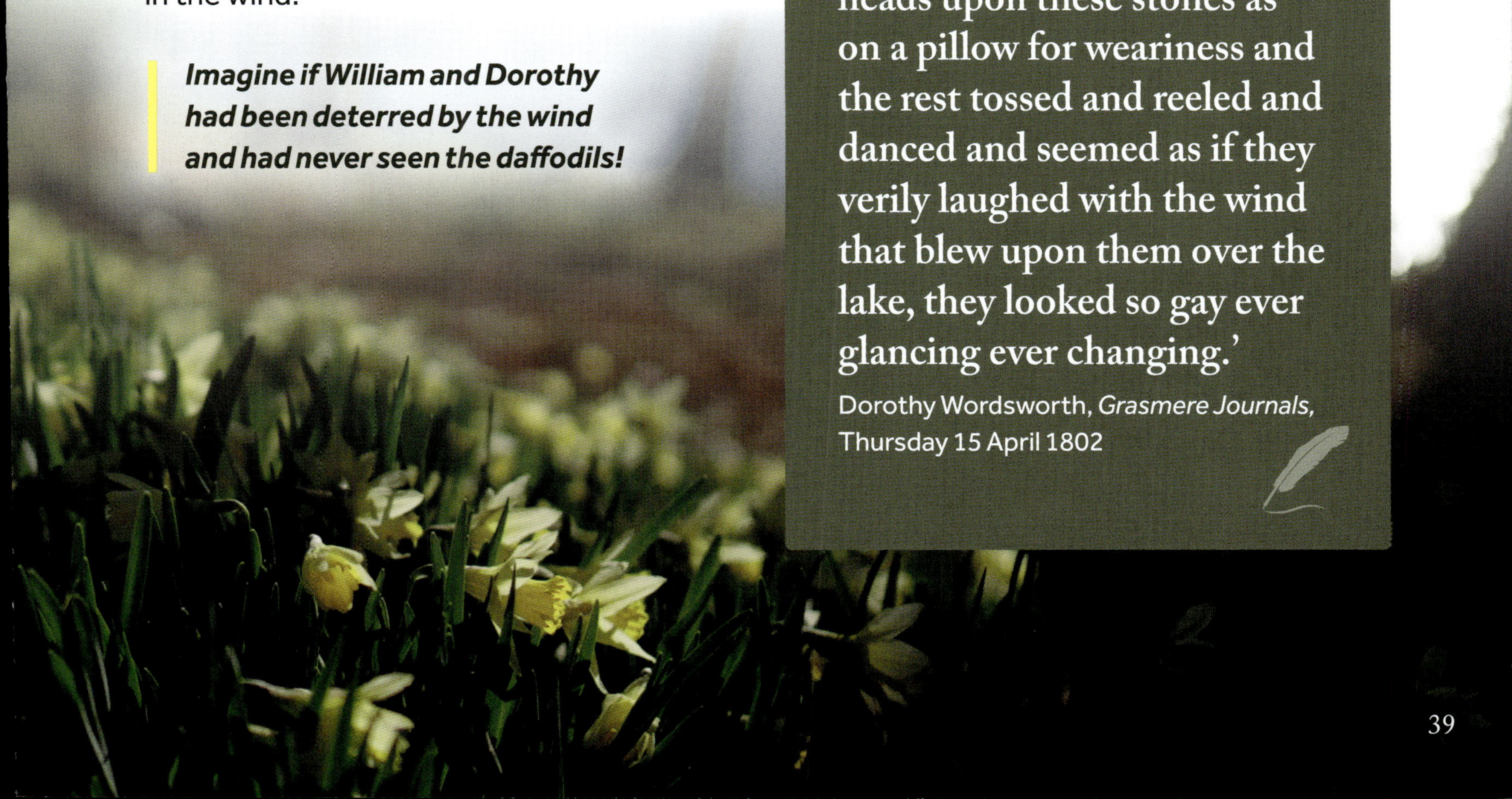

I wandered lonely as a cloud

After Dorothy and William returned home from Ullswater, Dorothy picked up her journal and wrote an account of their walk. Two years later, William read the description in Dorothy's journal, was reminded of the dancing daffodils, and was inspired to write a poem.

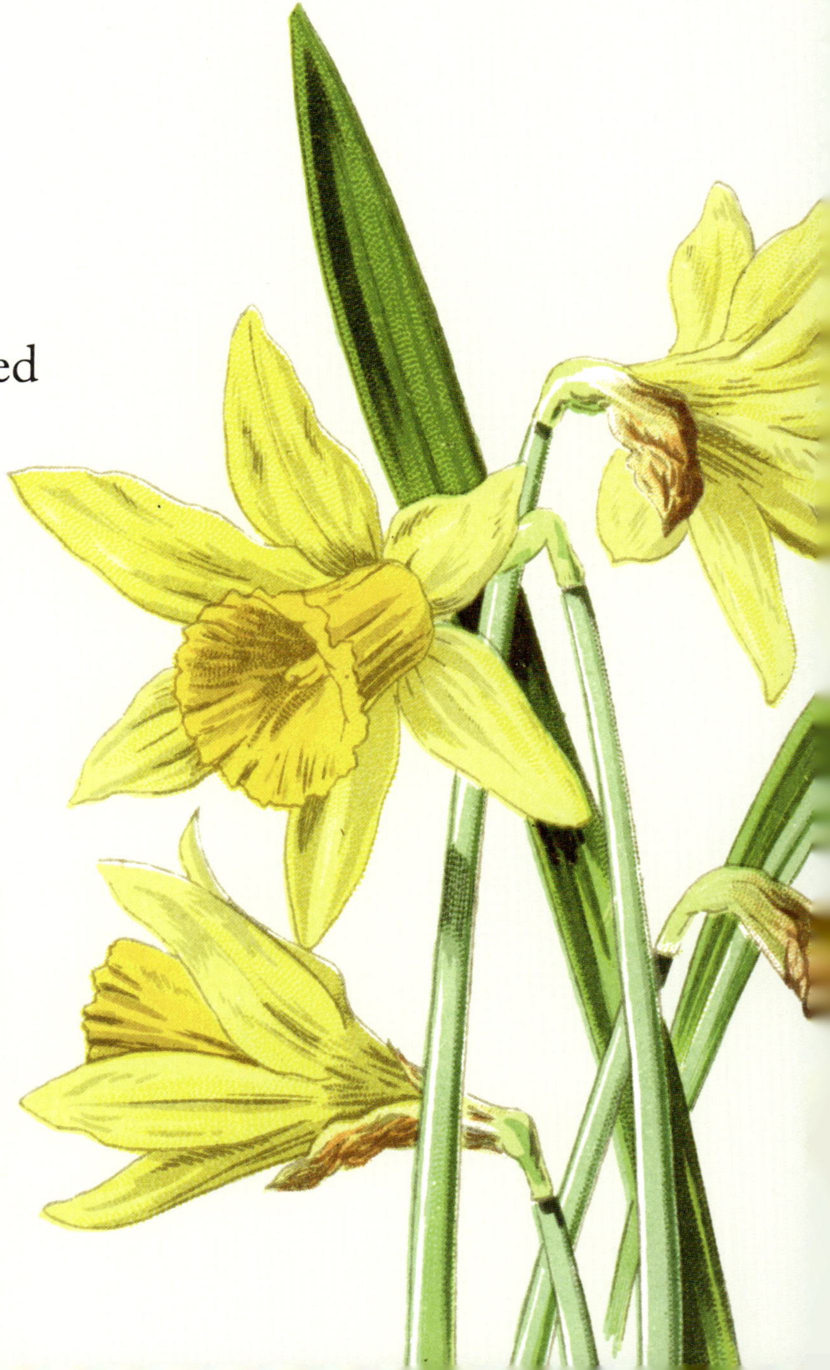

> ***'I wandered lonely as a cloud' is often said to be the most famous poem in the English language.***
>
> *If Dorothy had been too busy to write her journal that day, would William have written the poem?*

I wandered lonely as a cloud

William Wordsworth

1 I wandered lonely as a cloud
That floats on high o'er vales and hills,
When all at once I saw a crowd,
A host, of golden daffodils;
Beside the lake, beneath the trees,
Fluttering and dancing in the breeze.

2 Continuous as the stars that shine
And twinkle on the milky way,
They stretched in never-ending line
Along the margin of a bay:
Ten thousand saw I at a glance,
Tossing their heads in sprightly dance.

3 The waves beside them danced; but they
Out-did the sparkling waves in glee:
A poet could not but be gay,
In such a jocund company:
I gazed—and gazed—but little thought
What wealth the show to me had brought:

4 For oft, when on my couch I lie
In vacant or in pensive mood,
They flash upon that inward eye
Which is the bliss of solitude;
And then my heart with pleasure fills,
And dances with the daffodils.

Friends and strangers

Dorothy's life in Grasmere was far from solitary. Neighbours called for tea or supper and the Wordsworths visited them in return, exchanging news and gifts of plants and garden produce.

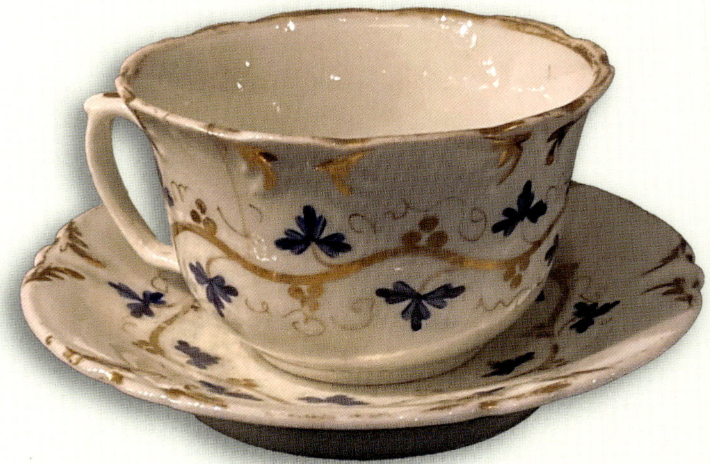

Teacup and saucer belonging to Dorothy Wordsworth

'Mr Simpson came in at dinner-time – drank tea with us and played at cards.'

Dorothy Wordsworth, *Grasmere Journals*, Saturday 24 October 1801

If you had been invited to tea with Dorothy at Dove Cottage, what gift would you have taken?

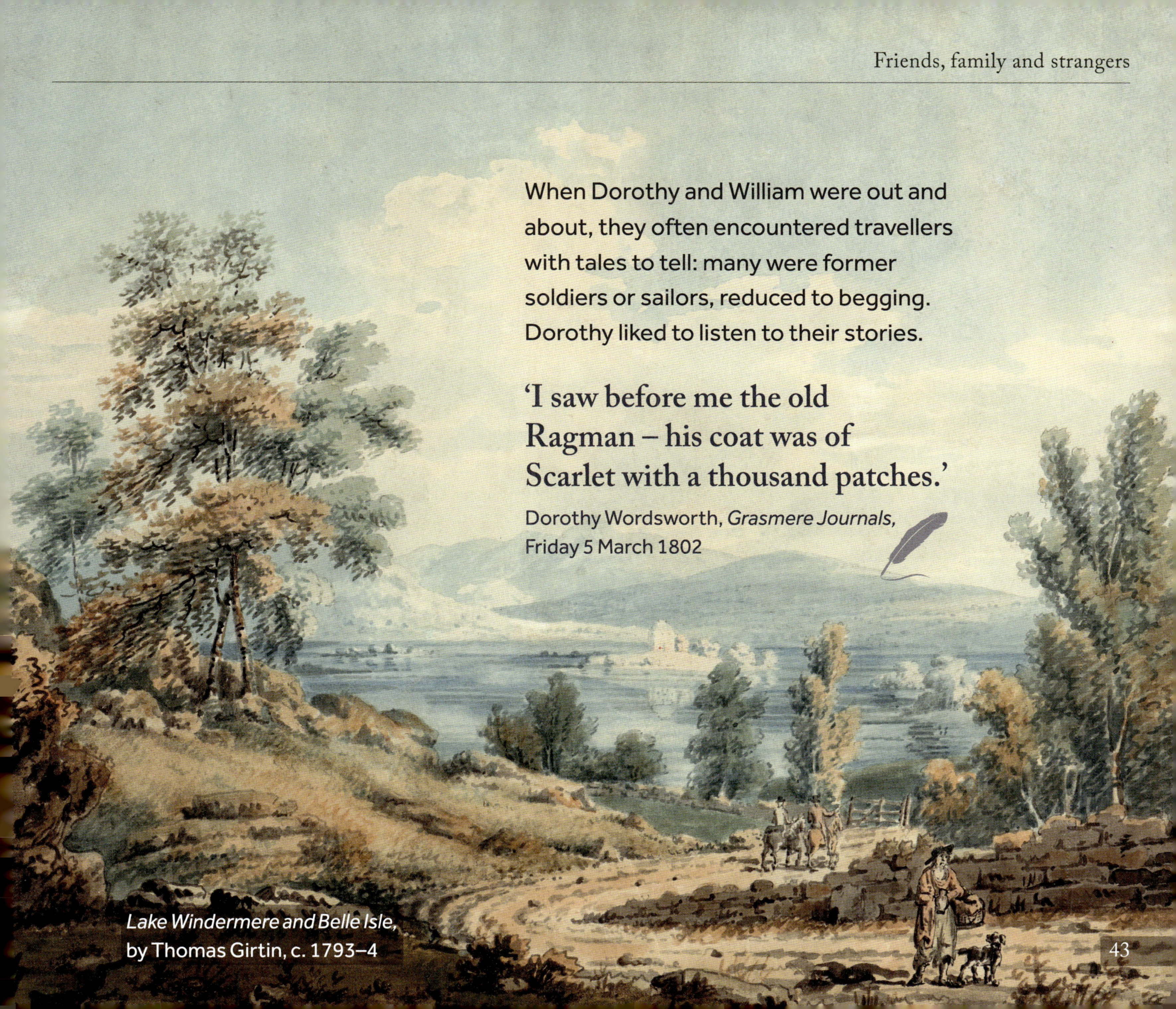

When Dorothy and William were out and about, they often encountered travellers with tales to tell: many were former soldiers or sailors, reduced to begging. Dorothy liked to listen to their stories.

'I saw before me the old Ragman – his coat was of Scarlet with a thousand patches.'

Dorothy Wordsworth, *Grasmere Journals,* Friday 5 March 1802

Lake Windermere and Belle Isle, by Thomas Girtin, c. 1793–4

Rain

Fine rain was good for the garden, but, more often than not, the Grasmere rain was heavy, or incessant, or both.

Wet days were a good opportunity to do indoor jobs, or to read by the fire, or to catch up on some sleep.

'So heavy a rain that I could not go for letters – put by the linen, mended stockings etc.'

Dorothy Wordsworth, *Grasmere Journals*, Friday 23 May 1800

What would you like to do, if it rains tomorrow?

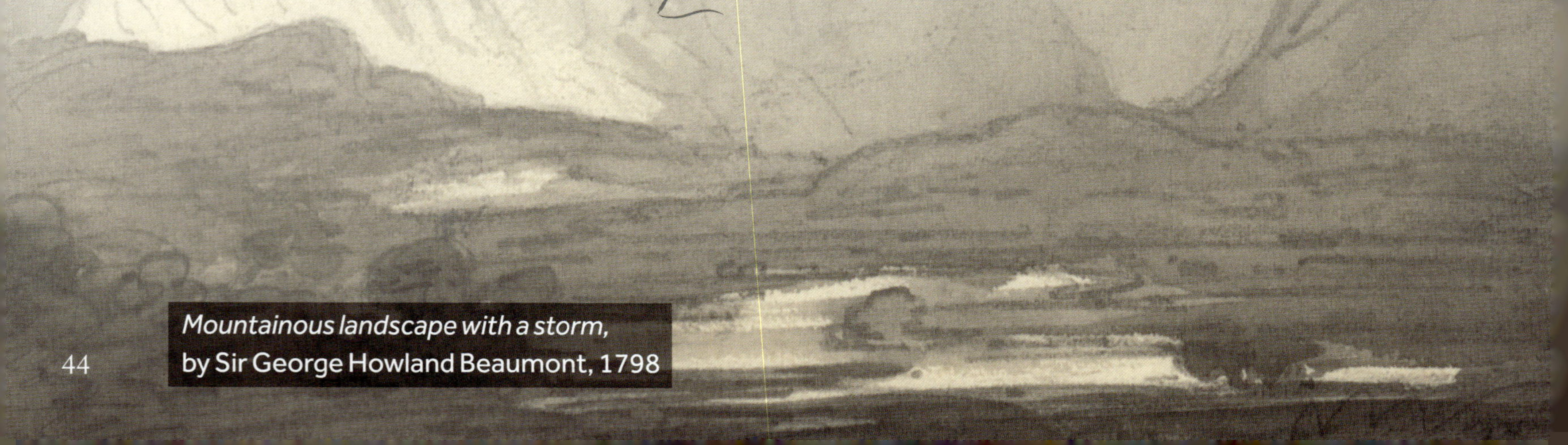

Mountainous landscape with a storm,
by Sir George Howland Beaumont, 1798

Cold feet, sore heads and toothache

Despite being such vigorous walkers, both Dorothy and William were often ill. Dorothy suffered badly from headaches and toothache; she also had trouble with her bowels.

A good sleep was usually the answer, but the Wordsworths also kept recipes for various home remedies to treat common ailments.

'We all went weary to bed. My Bowels very bad.'

Dorothy Wordsworth, *Grasmere Journals*, Monday 28 December 1801

A remedy for chilblains

1oz rosin
1oz beeswax
1os lard
2 spoonfuls sweet oil

To be simmered in a new pipkin*. The feet to be washed, a plaster of this mixture to be spread thinly & applied fresh every third night.

From the Wordsworths' Commonplace Book

*A pipkin was an earthenware pot that could be heated gently on the edge of the fire – good for making ointment

A new phase of life

On 4 October 1802 William Wordsworth married Mary Hutchinson, one of Dorothy's oldest and dearest friends. Their first child, John, was born in June 1803, and was followed by Dora, Thomas, Catharine and William junior.

Dorothy was a devoted aunt. Instead of making detailed observations of nature and the weather, Dorothy began to write about John's baby milestones: from his 'first inarticulate sounds' to his first steps.

'On Thursday the 14th April he first got up upon his feet by himself, with help of a stool. William wagered a guinea with me that he would walk in a fortnight.'

Dorothy Wordsworth, writing in the Wordsworths' Commonplace Book

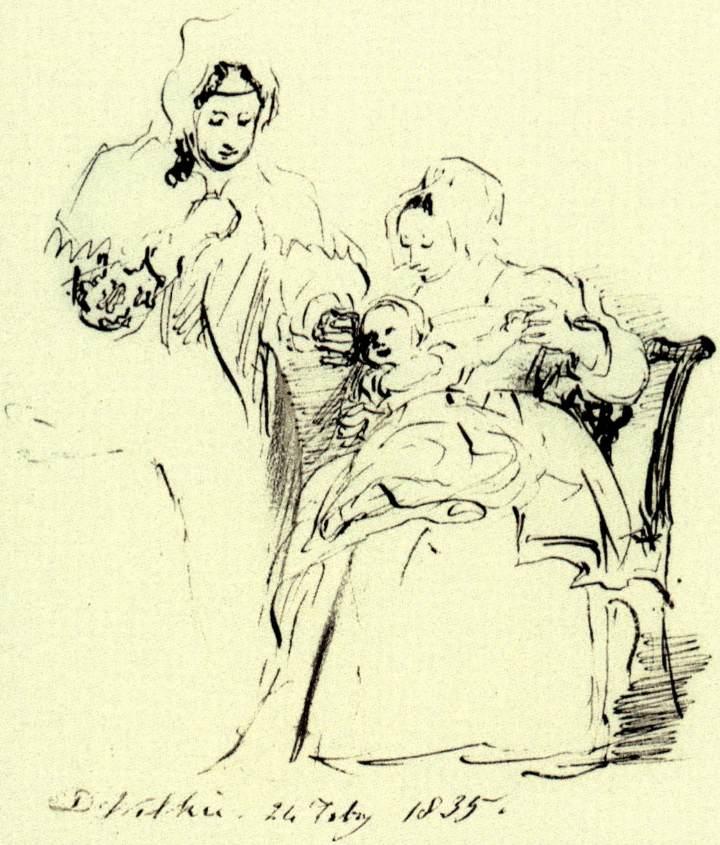

Sketch of two women with a baby, by Sir David Wilkie, 24 February 1835. From an album belonging to Dora Wordsworth.

The cottager to her infant

Dorothy Wordsworth

The days are cold, the nights are long,
The north-wind sings a doleful song;
Then hush again upon my breast;
All merry things are now at rest,
Save thee, my pretty Love!
The kitten sleeps upon the hearth,
The crickets long have ceased their mirth;
There's nothing stirring in the house
Save one wee, hungry, nibbling mouse,
Then why so busy thou?

What do you think inspired Dorothy to write this poem for her niece Dora?

Moving house

By 1808 the Wordsworths' little cottage was full to bursting.

The family moved to a new and bigger property on the other side of Grasmere, called Allan Bank. It was a cold house, with smoking chimneys, and it never felt like home. Two years later, they moved again, into the centre of the village.

Then life took a sad turn. First Catharine (nearly 4) and then Thomas (6) died. The family decided to move away, to the neighbouring hamlet of Rydal.

The house at Rydal Mount was spacious and comfortable, with a fine garden and views down to Rydal Water. It was very different from the little cottage in Grasmere but became a happy home.

> ***How do you suppose Dorothy felt when they had to keep moving house?***

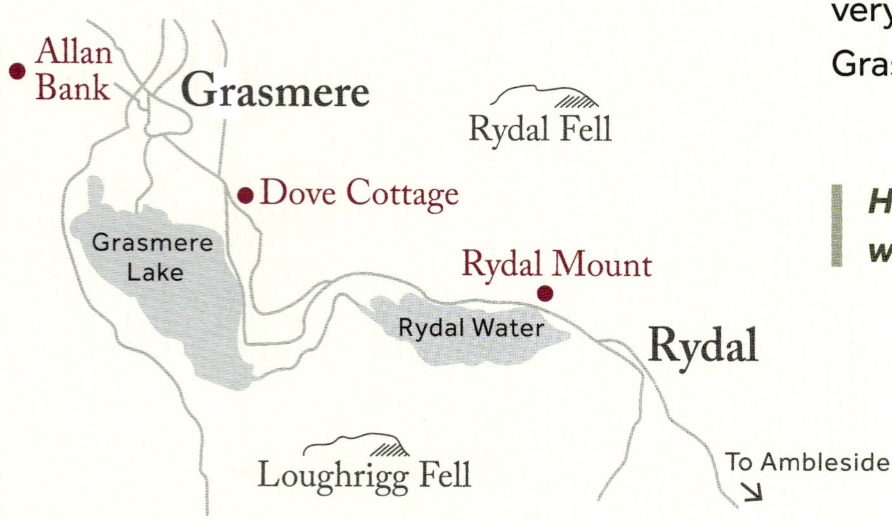

'William has taken a house at Rydale which is very pleasantly situated.'

Dorothy Wordsworth, Letter to
Richard Wordsworth, 11 January 1813

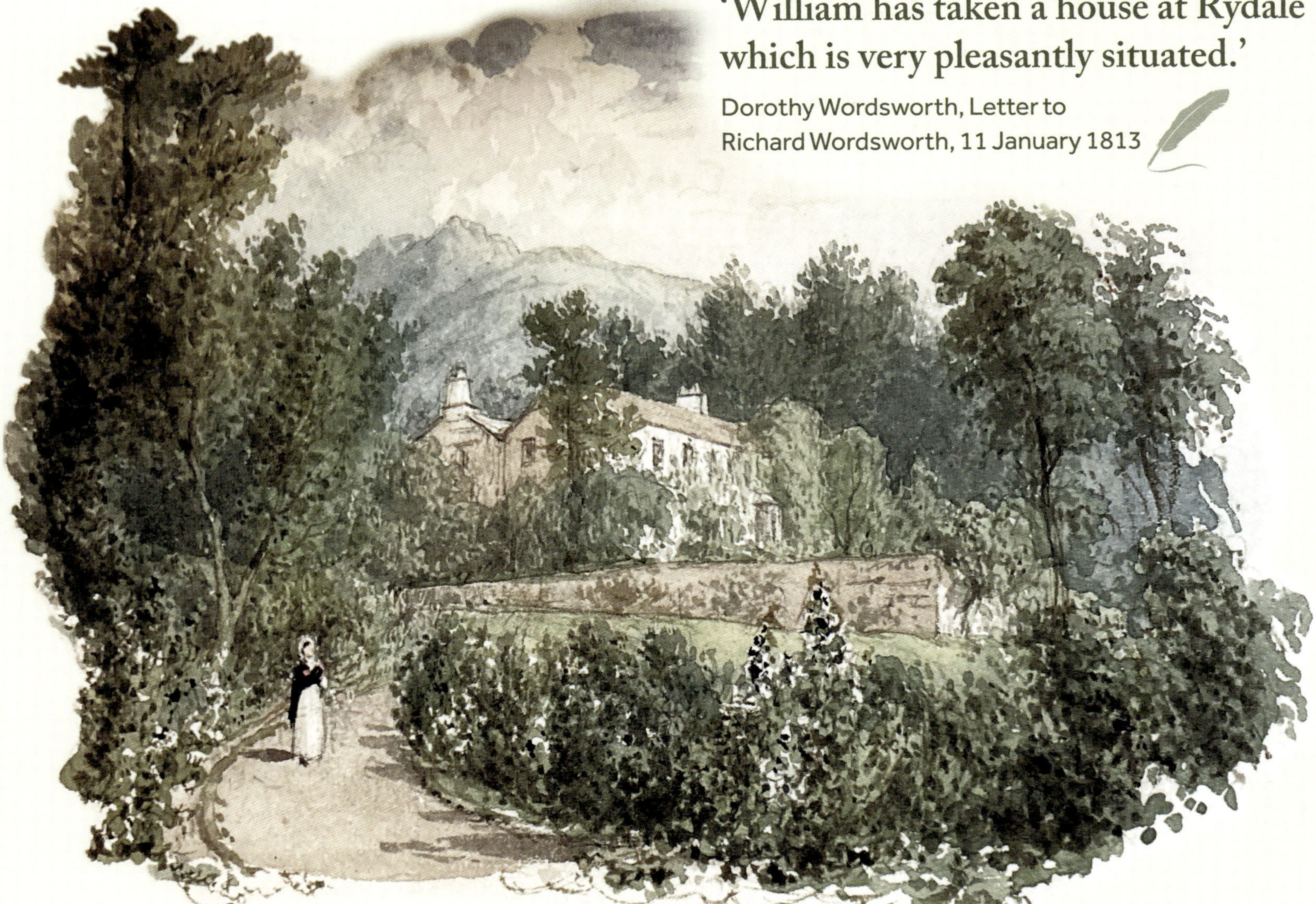

The Garden at Rydal Mount, by William Westall, 1831. From an album belonging to Dora Wordsworth.

After Grasmere

After moving to Rydal, Dorothy continued to care for the family as the Wordsworth children grew up and visitors came and went.

She continued to read, to transcribe William's poems, to walk and to keep in touch with friends.

Meanwhile, William's reputation as a poet spread far and wide. In 1843, he accepted the invitation of Queen Victoria to become Poet Laureate.

'I can walk as well as when but twenty years old, and can climb the hills better than in those days. The pure air of those places seems to restore all my youthful feelings.'

Dorothy Wordsworth, Letter to Robert Jones, 7 October 1825

What do you do to restore your youthful feelings?

From 1829 Dorothy began to experience bouts of serious illness. Several times she recovered, only to fall ill again. Now it was the turn of the family to care for her.

For the last two decades of her life Dorothy could no longer ramble about the hills. She continued to write, now and then, and still took an interest in the garden and the birds outside her window.

In 1850, her brother William died at the age of 80. Dorothy lived for another four years. She died peacefully at Rydal Mount, on 25 January 1855, aged 84.

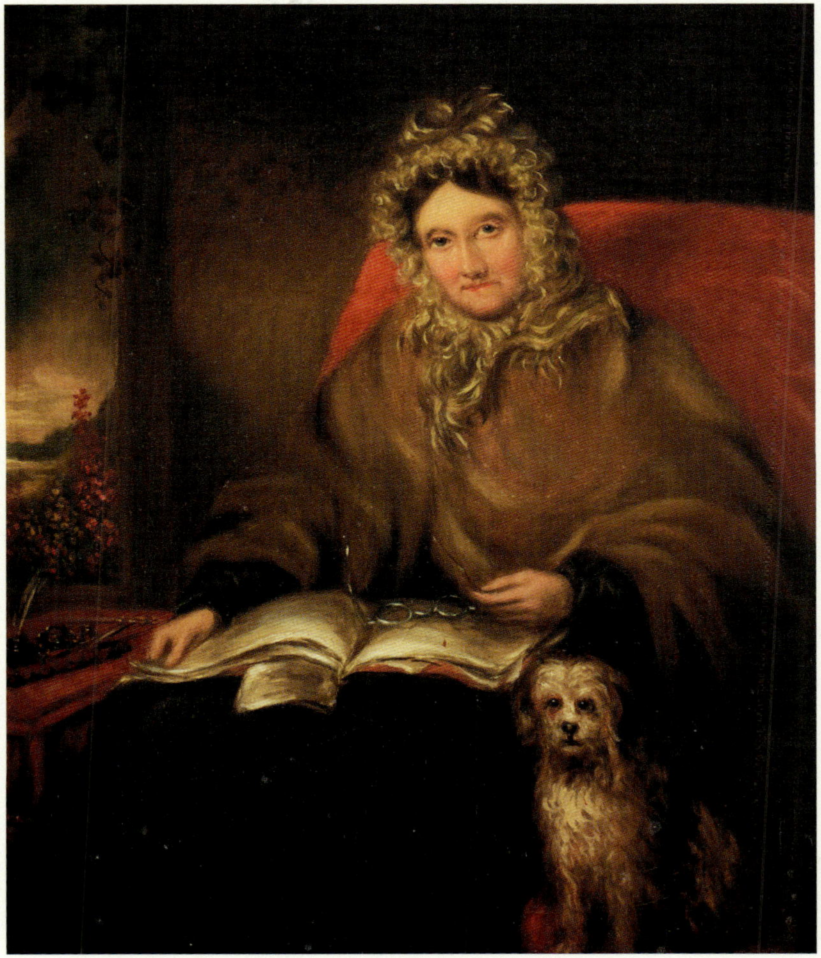

Portrait of Dorothy Wordsworth,
by Samuel Crosthwaite, 1833

Find out more

Places to visit

Dove Cottage in Grasmere, where the Wordsworths lived from December 1799–1808, is owned by the **Wordsworth Trust** and is open to the public all year round. The cottage, garden and orchard at Wordsworth Grasmere are wonderfully atmospheric, and the museum next door houses an extraordinary collection of manuscripts, books, paintings and personal items.

wordsworth.org.uk

wordsworth GRASMERE

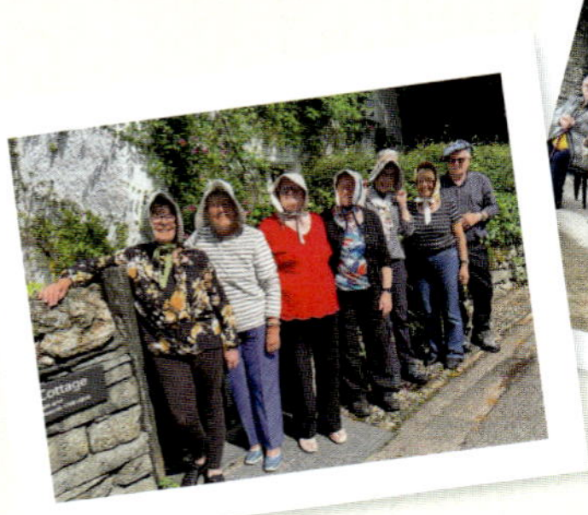

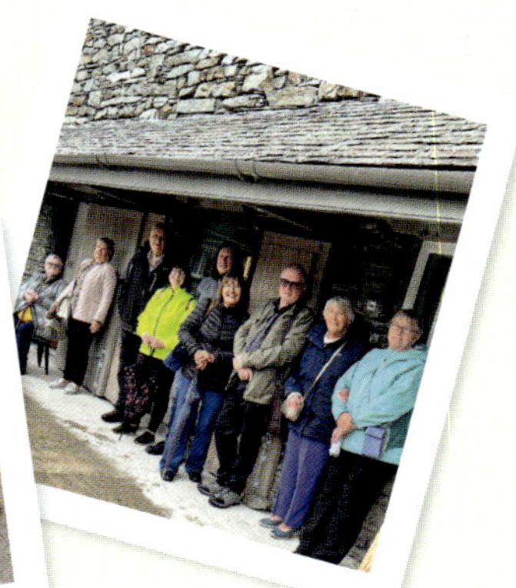

Wordsworth House in Cockermouth, where Dorothy and William were born, and **Allan Bank** where the family lived for two years after leaving Dove Cottage are both owned by the National Trust and well worth seeing.

nationaltrust.org.uk

Rydal Mount is the beautiful historic house where the Wordsworths lived from 1813 onwards and is still owned by descendants of the family. The house, gardens and tearoom are open for most of the year.

rydalmount.co.uk

Reading Dorothy

Dorothy Wordsworth's *Grasmere Journals* are widely available and very enjoyable to read. Many of her letters have also been published.

Dorothy Wordsworth – Wonders of the Everyday by Pamela Woof (published by the Wordsworth Trust, 2013) is a beautifully-written portrait of Dorothy's life, writings, friendships and travels.

Dorothy Wordsworth Walks

This free app created by the **Wordsworth Trust** includes walking routes to some of Dorothy's favourite places, with passages from her *Grasmere Journals* read by members of the Grasmere Women's Institute.

wordsworth.org.uk/dorothy-wordsworth-walks

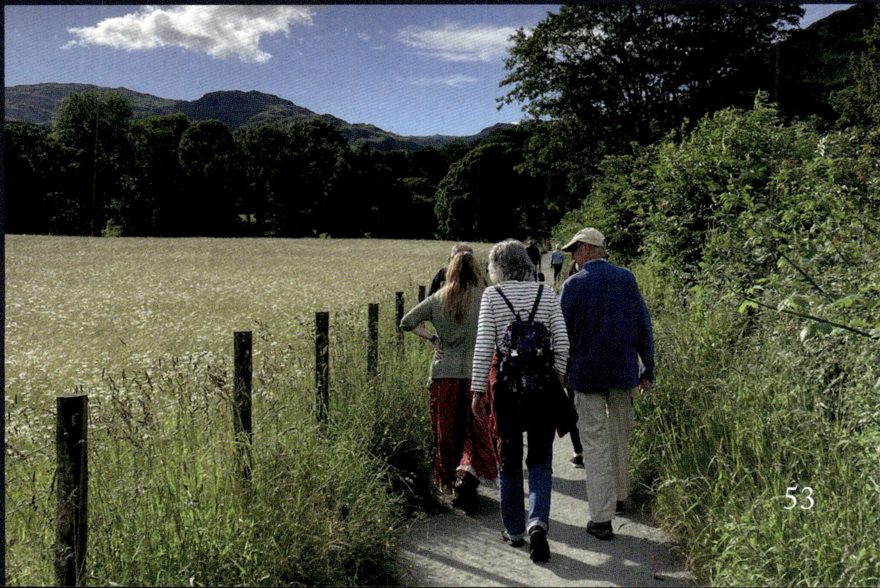

About Open Ended Books

Open Ended Books is the dementia-friendly publishing imprint of Equal Arts. Our aim is to enable people living with early to moderate dementia to continue reading for pleasure. We create beautiful and life-affirming books designed to stimulate the imagination and support conversation and shared reading with friends and family members. Our approach is informed by people with personal experience of dementia, and health and care professionals.

'Reading for pleasure is good for brain health because it reduces stress, keeps the mind active and improves mood. Titles from Open Ended Books can support people living with dementia by reducing the cognitive load associated with longer texts and complex narratives, enabling them to enjoy reading for longer.'

Dr Karen Franks, Consultant in Old Age Psychiatry at Gateshead Health NHS Foundation Trust

To find out more please **scan this QR code** or go to **equalarts.org.uk/dementia-friendly-reading**

Open Ended Books

About Equal Arts

Equal Arts is a leading creative ageing charity supporting older people and those living with dementia.

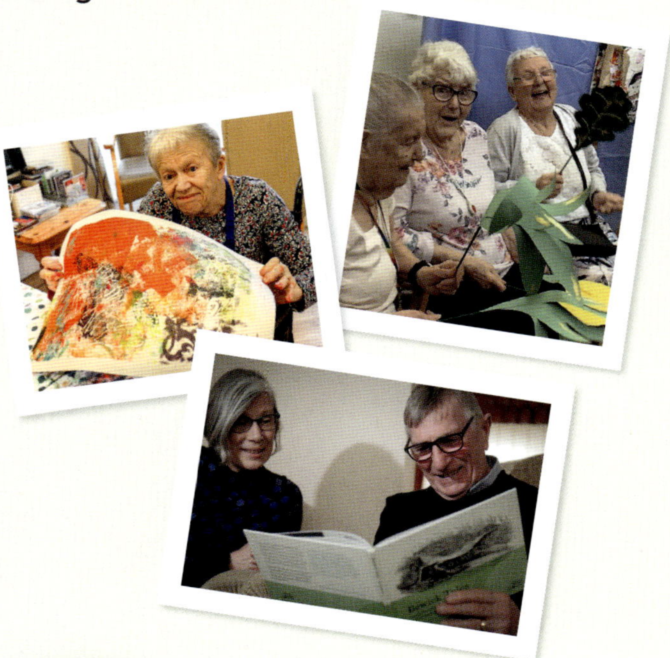

equal arts

Improving older people's lives through creativity

Our artist-led creative programmes provide opportunities to improve wellbeing and reduce loneliness. We work across artforms with visual artists, musicians, theatre practitioners, writers and curators, providing opportunities for people to explore their imagination and live in the moment.

About the author

Sarah Lawrance leads on dementia-friendly reading and publishing at Equal Arts. She loves working with people and heritage collections to create stories.

Acknowledgements

Equal Arts is extremely grateful to the Wordsworth Trust for supporting the research and development of this book and for providing images of objects in their collection. We would especially like to thank Jeff Cowton, Melissa Mitchell, Victoria Mitchell, and Rebecca Turner for their patience, kindness and thoughtful feedback on early drafts.

We would like to thank our readers David Foster, Anita Goundry, Julia Green, Mike and Liz Smith and Gill Taylor for their insightful comments, and our book designer Wendy Lewis for her painstaking work and creativity.

Finally, we are grateful to Newcastle Libraries for sharing our commitment to dementia-friendly reading and to the Dulverton Trust and Garfield Weston for contributions to our core funding which have helped to make this publication possible.

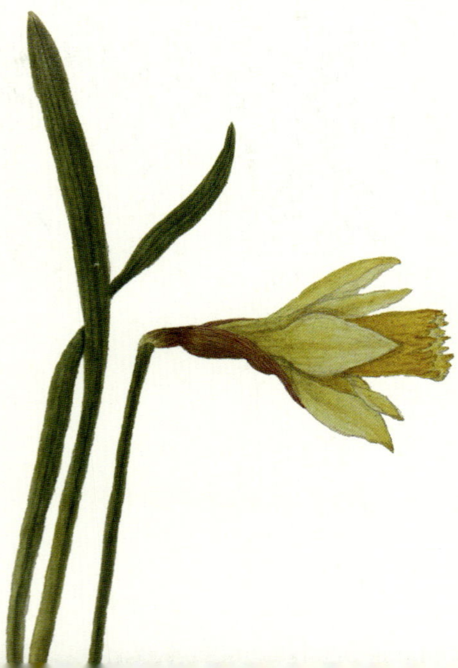

Picture credits

Except where stated below, the images in this book depict objects in the Wordsworth Trust collection and are used by kind permission.

We are also grateful for the following images and permissions:

Page 4: portrait of a young woman and Page 51: portrait of Dorothy Wordsworth by Samuel Crosthwaite; reproduced from images in the collection at Rydal Mount and used by permission of the owners; with thanks to Walker Ellis Associates photography.

Page 8: horse and carriage – illustration from a book by typefounder Vincent Figgins, dated 1836. With thanks to Graham Williams.

Pages 14, 17 and 27: interior views of Dove Cottage – photos by G. Gardner.

Page 15: woman hanging out washing, Page 26: swallow and house martin, Page 30: thrush and Page 32: pike; illustrations by Thomas Bewick, reproduced from books in the Pease collection at Newcastle Libraries.

Page 18: man and woman sitting at a table, by John Harden, 1805. Copyright Abbot Hall Art Gallery/ Bridgeman Images.

Page 22: foxglove and Page 56 wild daffodil, reproduced from watercolours in the Collinson collection at Newcastle Libraries, artist/s unknown.

Page 32: silhouette of Dorothy walking – artwork by Alex Jakob Whitworth.

Pages 38–39: wild daffodils at Ullswater – photograph by Street Films.

Page 40: 19th-century illustration of daffodils – photograph by iStock.com/ Ivan Burmistrov.

Other photographs supplied by Equal Arts and the Wordsworth Trust.

Open Ended Books

Published by Open Ended Books, 2025

Open Ended Books is the publishing imprint of Equal Arts.

Equal Arts is a registered charity no. 517352.

Postal address:
Equal Arts,
Newcastle City Library,
33 New Bridge Street,
Newcastle upon Tyne NE1 8AX

Website:
www.equalarts.org.uk/open-ended-books

Author: Sarah Lawrance

Design: Wendy Lewis

ISBN 978-1-7385229-1-0

A CIP catalogue record for this book is available from the British Library.

Printing arranged by Biddles in association with Carbon Neutral Climate Partner manufacturers.

Print product with financial
climate contribution
ClimatePartner.com/18507-2401-1007

Produced using FSC and PEFC certified materials.